Adult ADHD

A Comprehensive Guide to Attention Deficit Hyperactivity Disorder in Adults

Table of Contents

Introduction

Thank you for taking the time to pick up this book on adult ADHD.

This book covers the topic of Attention Deficit Hyperactivity Disorder in adults, and aims to serve as a comprehensive guide to the disorder. In the following chapters, you will learn about how ADHD is diagnosed, what the different types of ADHD are, the common symptoms that people experience, the different pharmaceutical drugs that are commonly prescribed to combat ADHD, as well as some alternative therapies that have been used.

Many people associate ADHD with children, but ADHD can also continue in to adulthood. Oftentimes, the symptoms experienced by adults differ slightly from those experienced as children. These symptoms can present a range of challenges in the workplace, in relationships, and in the sufferer's personal life.

This book provides a range of strategies that are commonly used to combat these symptoms and provides practical strategies for lessening the effect that ADHD can have on a person's relationships, and career.

Please remember that this book is not intended to be medical advice. It simply aims to serve as an overview of ADHD in adults, detailing the many ways that ADHD is regularly treated. Before beginning any treatment plan, or taking any medication, always consult with a medical professional to assess your personal situation.

Once again, thanks for choosing this book, I hope you find it to be helpful!

Chapter 1 – What is ADHD?

You have likely heard quite a lot about Attention Deficit Hyperactivity Disorder (ADHD) in recent years. You see it mentioned in television shows, movies, radio, and on social media. It seems as if more and more people are being diagnosed with ADHD. It's hard to tell if the prevalence of ADHD is actually increasing, or if simply more people are seeking a diagnosis for their children's behavioral issues.

Most researchers report that the number of school-age children who have ADHD could be anywhere from 5% to 8% of the total population of school-age kids. The Center for Disease Control (CDC), on the other hand, pins the number at a whopping 11% of all school-age children.

The trouble is that it can be rather difficult to accurately diagnose ADHD. As a result, many people are misdiagnosed with this condition.

Many doctors have mistakenly labeled a child as having ADHD, but in truth, they may actually have a separate learning, behavioral, or mental deficiency. On the other hand, there might also be some kids who actually have the disorder, but they have not received a proper diagnosis for it. What many people do not realize is, ADHD can actually overlap with other mental health issues, making it hard to identify.

What experts all agree on is that Attention Deficiency Hyperactivity Disorder is one of the most common mental disorders in children; this is according to both the National Institute of Mental Health and the Center for Disease Control. It's so heavily associated with children in fact, that many people don't realize that ADHD can actually exist in adulthood.

ADHD Through the Years

There is a misconception, particularly among older generations, that Attention Deficit Hyperactivity Disorder is a "modern problem", and that it "did not exist" back in their day. The same people point to the fact that the number of American children diagnosed with ADHD has increased by a whopping 42% between the years 2003 and 2011. At first glance, those numbers seem to prove the argument of the older folks. But what do these numbers really mean? Do they indicate that more people have the condition now than a decade ago, or simply that more people are seeking diagnosis? It's a complex question to answer.

The truth is, people are now more aware of ADHD, more research is being done on the subject, and there are now a range of accurate assessment tools to diagnose people with ADHD. In short, doctors are now more aware of ADHD and they also understand the disorder much better, which allows them to better detect it.

ADHD Around the Country and Around the World

Here's another conundrum related to ADHD; why does it seem that rates vary depending on the location? Why is it that more than 13% of children in Alabama, Kentucky, Arkansas, Rhode Island, South Carolina, and Ohio have been diagnosed with ADHD, while other states like Colorado, California, and Nevada only report 7% or lower?

Why is there such a huge difference? Most experts have concluded that there might not be enough properly-trained mental health professionals in certain places, which is why the kids there could not get a proper diagnosis. There is also a chance that the parents in areas with low instances of ADHD do not want to have their children diagnosed.

The discrepancy gets even bigger when you look at it on a global scale. For instance, surveys found that 11% of Australian kids have one form or another of ADHD, while in the United Kingdom, only 3% of the children had it.

These numbers are actually very misleading as health care providers from different countries might be using different criteria for diagnosing ADHD. There are also the cultural factors, social stigma, and economic issues (cost of testing and treatment) that need to be considered in order to make an accurate estimate of the actual number of people who have ADHD.

ADHD in Boys vs Girls

One of the misconceptions that many people have about ADHD is that it is a male-only condition. Currently, boys are twice as likely to get an ADHD diagnosis as girls, but these statistics might start to shift once researchers shed more light on how ADHD presents itself in females.

There are three types of ADHD: the inattentive, the hyperactive-impulsive, and a combination of the first two. Girls with ADHD are more likely to manifest the symptoms of being inattentive ADHD sufferers rather than being the hyperactive type. The inattentive type is much harder to diagnose, which could explain the difference in ADHD prevalence between women and men.

ADHD in Adults

Being a normal, responsible adult is hard enough, but when you find that you are constantly late for your appointments, you have trouble getting organized, you tend to forget important things, and you regularly feel overwhelmed with all of the responsibilities that you have, there's a good chance that you may have adult ADHD.

It is not just children that can be affected by ADHD. There are many adults who are also living with ADHD today, most of them undiagnosed. This disorder has a wide range of symptoms that can negatively affect most adults' careers and personal relationships.

Fortunately, if you have adult ADHD, there are things that you can do to get help, and simply learning more about the disorder is the very first step to managing your symptoms. Once you understand the challenges of ADHD, then you will learn to compensate for your weaknesses, and take advantage of the strengths that ADHD can provide.

Understanding Adult Attention Deficit Hyperactivity Disorder

What is it?

ADHD is when a person shows a consistent pattern of inattention and/or hyperactivity that negatively affects his/her productivity or development.

Inattention is when the person suddenly wanders away from their tasks to do other things that are irrelevant. This kind of person lacks persistence, cannot seem to focus, and is almost always disorganized. Those who do not understand ADHD seem to think that these behaviors are due to the person being defiant, or lazy, but that is not the case at all.

On the other hand, hyperactivity means that the person cannot stop themselves from fidgeting. Adults with ADHD will seem constantly restless, which can wear other people out because they can't seem to sit still.

With hyperactivity almost always comes impulsivity. This means that the person often makes hasty decisions without thinking about them first. These people desire immediate gratification, and they are also (unintentionally) socially intrusive, often interrupting others. If you have adult ADHD, the problem really becomes serious when you start making important decisions without thinking them through.

To give you an idea on whether you might have ADHD or not, here are some of the common signs to look out for:

10 Signs of Inattentive ADHD

1. You get easily distracted – Your mind tends to wander off somewhere whenever you are bored, like when you are in a board meeting, or if someone is explaining something to you at length. Sometimes you daydream because you are bored, and sometimes, even when you are trying your hardest to concentrate, you still seem to get distracted by every little thing.

2. You have trouble paying attention to details – There are times when your work is impeccable, but when your ADHD kicks in, your work is riddled with mistakes. This gives other people the impression that you are not putting enough effort into your work, or that you are not trying in the first place.

3. You are disorganized – You might have ADHD if you find it difficult to keep your environment clean and organized. When you peek inside your purse, how many items are crammed in there? Do you even know the exact contents of your bag? Do you always seem to miss important appointments?

4. You have difficulty managing your time – When you have ADHD, it will seem as if time flows differently for you. You are often late for important appointments. You also like to leave things until the last minute, which means pulling an all-nighter is something that you are very familiar with.

5. You have poor memory – Not only do you have trouble remembering important dates, there are also

times when you might not know what day of the week it is.

6. It is a constant struggle for you to complete tasks – You do not have any trouble starting a task, it is finishing it that you have a problem with. When you start working, you start strong, but you cannot seem to maintain your momentum and motivation to see it all the way until the end.

7. You avoid tasks – If you have tasks at hand, you tend to easily convince yourself to procrastinate. Unless the deadline is just around the corner, you struggle to convince yourself to start working.

8. You always seem uninterested – Do people often accuse you of not listening? If you have ADHD, you may find it hard to look people directly in the eye when you are having a conversation, which gives the impression that you are not interested in what they have to say.

9. You tend to lose concentration when driving – Here is where ADHD can become really dangerous. You sometimes get bored while driving on the highway and get distracted by even the slightest thing, like a funny shaped cloud, or that curious piece of paper on the floor.

10. You find mundane tasks difficult – You find doing basic domestic tasks like doing the laundry, going grocery shopping, making a doctor's appointment, and many other mundane everyday tasks quite difficult.

10 Signs of Hyperactive-Impulsive ADHD

1. You are always moving – You like to have a full schedule, and you do not like any kind of downtime. People often mistake you for being younger than your actual age as you always seem to have a lot of energy.

2. You cannot sit still for extended periods – Even back when you were a kid, you had trouble sitting still and you also probably liked to jump around the house causing all sorts of trouble. Now that you are an adult, you learned to sit still, but you still fidget in your chair, tap your foot, fiddle with your pen, and other kinds of movements.

3. You cannot help interrupt others when they are speaking – Because your brain is always working on overdrive, you tend to finish other people's sentences. There are also times when you actually interrupt others while speaking because you are afraid that you might forget what you want to say if you do not say it immediately.

4. You like to talk a lot – Your family and friends know that you are very talkative, and they always remind you of the fact. You are also the type of person who likes to talk loudly, and you just love to debate with others.

5. You do not like to wait – Waiting for an extended period is a challenge for you. Whenever you are forced to wait, like when you are in line at the bank, waiting for your friend to arrive to meet you for coffee, or even waiting for the pizza you ordered to arrive, you always feel impatient, bored, and restless.

6. You drive fast – You are always in a hurry, even if you are early for your appointment. You find yourself

constantly speeding down the road, and likely have an extensive collection of speeding tickets.

7. You are not fond of slowness – You get impatient whenever you are stuck behind "slow" people. When you ask for something, you want it done yesterday. You tend to speed through tasks just so you do not have to deal with slow people.

8. You feel "internal restlessness" – Whenever you are required to stand or sit really still, like when you are going through a medical examination, you feel very uncomfortable.

9. You make quick decisions – There are times when a quick decision is good. However, quick and harsh decisions are often counterproductive. You do not have the patience to think things through before you make a decision.

10. You say things on impulse – You often offend other people because you tend to say what is on your mind without thinking if you are hurting other people's feelings.

What Causes ADHD?

ADHD usually starts to manifest during childhood and is considered as a developmental disorder. For many people, the symptoms seem to slowly disappear before adulthood, but for some the condition will persist.

Although scientists are not completely sure as to what causes ADHD, they believe that it is influenced by the person's genes, their environment, and the hardwiring of their brain. If you have gotten a diagnosis of ADHD when you were a kid, chances are that you have taken at least some of the symptoms with you into adulthood.

The sad part about this disorder is that it often goes unrecognized. This was not extremely prevalent in the past, because very few people were aware of ADHD, and even fewer actually understood what it was. Back then, instead of finding the real issue, everyone (your family, friends, teachers, etc.) labeled you as a dreamer, a slacker, a troublemaker, or simply, as just a bad student.

When you were younger, you might have been able to cover up or compensate for the symptoms of ADHD. However, now that you're an adult with more responsibilities, your symptoms can start to cause real issues. In adulthood there are more balls that you have to juggle, like your career, your family, keeping a clean household, and your social life. For a regular person, this is already a tall order, but for someone who has ADHD, this can feel impossible to manage.

In order to receive a proper diagnosis of ADHD as an adult, you need to have:

- Several symptoms apparent before age 12

- At least five symptoms of either inattention and/or hyperactivity impulsivity.

- Symptoms that are present in at least two settings. For instance, in the home and at work/school.

- Evidence that the symptoms are interfering with your functioning in said settings.

- Signs of other mental health conditions that usually occur with ADHD, like conduct disorder, anxiety, and/or depression.

Getting a professional diagnosis is not as easy as getting your blood tested or taking a test online. You need to get a detailed evaluation by a trained health professional who is actually trained and experienced in dealing with ADHD. After the evaluation, the medical professional will check if you fit into the criteria of ADHD according to the guidelines of the Diagnostic and Statistical Manual of Mental Disorders, which is the official diagnostic guide book used in the United States.

You will be answering questionnaires, and the physician will also use rating scales, interviews, intellectual screenings, and others to ensure that you do actually have ADHD. The symptoms of ADHD can look a lot like those of other serious mental conditions such as depression, bipolar disorder, sleep problems, learning disabilities, and many more. This is why extensive and detailed testing needs to be made so that the medical professional can determine if you do have ADHD, an entirely different condition, or ADHD and a co-existing mental condition.

In addition, the latest edition of the DSM takes into account how the different symptoms manifest in adults as compared to children. This is very important as many symptoms of adult ADHD were overlooked in the previous editions of the DSM.

How Does ADHD Affect Adults?

Many, if not most of the adults who actually have ADHD may not even know they have it. These adults can feel like it is impossible for them to get organized, they cannot stick to one job, and they have trouble remembering even the most important appointments. Even mundane daily tasks such as getting up in the morning, preparing to go to work, being productive, and so on can be very challenging for someone who has undiagnosed ADHD.

For those who think that ADHD is just a simple ailment that makes people easily distracted, there are actually a lot of serious consequences that come along with it. People with undiagnosed ADHD are usually those who:

- Have problems at work

- Have had numerous failed relationships

- Have a history of academic problems

- Have a long history of traffic accidents and violations

Just like teens who have ADHD, adult ADHD sufferers also like to multi-task; they like to do several things at once to be "more productive" which usually is never the case as they typically fail to finish any of the tasks they start. Most of the people who have ADHD prefer using "quick fixes" rather than taking all the prerequisite steps to achieve greater and better rewards.

Other reasons why a person may not have been diagnosed with ADHD until well into their adult life are:

- Their family or teachers failed to recognize the signs early on.

- They may have just a mild form of ADHD.

- They only began to be affected by their symptoms when faced with the responsibilities of adulthood.

However, it is not uncommon for young adults with undiagnosed ADHD to have a lot of trouble with their studies during college, because the classes required intense concentration.

If left untreated, ADHD in adults can lead to many problems, but it is never too late to recognize, diagnose, and treat this disorder along with any other mental condition that might have come with it. With effective treatment, sufferers of adult ADHD can lead normal and productive lives.

Adult ADHD and Women

Women are more likely to have inattentive ADHD, which means that their symptoms were likely to be overlooked when they were children. If a child often daydreams and is disorganized, it is typically dismissed as a character flaw, rather than digging deeper to find out that it may actually be ADHD. This is the reason why many women and some men are diagnosed as having inattentive ADHD later in life.

Women can also have hyperactive-impulsive ADHD, but the cases are few and far between.

You have an increased risk of having ADHD if:

- You have an immediate family member, like a parent or a sibling, that has ADHD or other mental health disorders.

- Your mother drank and smoked when she was pregnant with you.

- You were exposed to environmental toxins, like lead, which was found in the paint and pipes of older houses and buildings.

- You were born ahead of term.

Now for some good news, you can beat the challenges imposed upon you by ADHD. You might feel overwhelmed by all of the symptoms, but with knowledge, a good support system, and some creativity, you can manage the symptoms of ADHD instead of letting them dictate how you should lead your life.

The Most Common Myths About Adult ADHD

Myth – ADHD is just an excuse for not having enough willpower. People who say they have ADHD can focus on things that they find interesting, so they should be able to do the same with other things if they really wanted to.

Fact – Although ADHD looks like simply a lack of willpower, it is actually very different. ADHD is essentially an imbalance of the chemical makeup of the brain which affects its management systems.

Myth – ADHD sufferers can never pay attention when needed.

Fact – It is a well-known fact that people with ADHD can give their full concentration to activities that they genuinely enjoy doing. However, they cannot do the same with boring, repetitive tasks; their mind will start to wander and cause them to lose focus just minutes into a task that they do not like doing.

Myth – Everyone has symptoms of ADHD, and if you are smart and disciplined enough you can overcome them.

Fact – ADHD can affect people of different levels of intelligence. Even though everyone may sometimes show symptoms of ADHD, only those who have chronic impairments due to these symptoms are given a professional ADHD diagnosis. Overcoming these symptoms is not simply a matter of intelligence or discipline.

Myth – You cannot have ADHD and depression, anxiety, and other mental disorders at the same time.

Fact – The truth is that people with ADHD are six times more likely to suffer from other mental ailments.

Myth – Unless you were diagnosed with ADHD as a child, you cannot have it as an adult.

Fact – A lot of adults have struggled for most of their lives because they had unrecognized and undiagnosed ADHD. A large number of ADHD cases go undiagnosed, as evidenced by the differing rates of diagnosis between cities and countries.

Complications Brought About by Adult ADHD

ADHD can really make your life difficult because it is linked to:

- Poor performance in school and at work.

- Constantly being unemployed because of poor work performance.

- Being frequently involved in car accidents

- A higher likelihood of being an alcoholic or addicted to other substances.

- Difficulties in maintaining any kind of personal relationship with others.

- Being in poor physical and mental health.

- Having very low self-esteem.

- Depression and suicidal thoughts.

- Coexisting mental conditions that are left untreated.

Although ADHD will not directly cause you to have other mental or educational problems, there are other conditions that regularly occur alongside ADHD, which can make both the diagnosis and the treatment a whole lot more difficult.

Some of the accompanying mental disorders include:

Mood disorders – Mood disorders such as depression, bipolar disorder, and borderline personality disorder often accompany adult ADHD. Although mood problems are not directly tied to ADHD, suffering through a repeated pattern of discouraging and frustrating failures can make them worse.

Anxiety – Adults with ADHD are often also diagnosed as having anxiety disorders. When you have anxiety, it will cause you to have overwhelming worries, nervousness, and a mess of other symptoms. In short, if you have anxiety, your ADHD can make it much worse than it should be.

Other mental illnesses – When you are an adult with previously undiagnosed ADHD, then you are more prone to other psychiatric disorders, like personality disorders, intermittent explosive disorder, and you are also very much at risk of substance abuse.

Learning disabilities – Adults with previously undiagnosed ADHD often scored lower than their peers on academic tests. Learning disabilities include having trouble with comprehension, and problems in communicating.

Chapter 2 – What are the Symptoms of Adult ADHD?

As of now, there is still no singular means of testing individuals for ADHD, however, a qualified mental health care professional or a psychiatrist can do a diagnostic evaluation to determine if the patient indeed shows signs of ADHD. These healthcare professionals draw their information from reliable sources like the ADHD symptom checklist, standardized behavior rating scales, the history of mental health of the patient, and any information gathered from the family members or friends who know the patient quite well. Some health professionals might even conduct cognitive ability testing, and ask for academic achievements just to rule out the possibility of learning disabilities.

Do keep in mind that a single, brief office observation is not enough to come up with an ADHD diagnosis, nor does talking with the examiner alone. For one thing, the patient might not be exhibiting any of the symptoms of ADHD during his/her visit to the clinic, and besides, the physician needs an extensive medical and personal history of the patient to come to a definite conclusion. Diagnosing ADHD requires the consideration of the possible presence of co-existing medical conditions.

The clinical guidelines used to diagnose ADHD in both adults and children can be found in the Diagnostic and Statistical Manual of Mental Disorders, 5th edition, which is provided by the American Psychiatric Association. These are the same set of guidelines that are used in most research and clinical practices.

During the evaluation process, the psychiatric professional will endeavor to determine the gravity of the symptoms that have manifested in the adult, and if the same symptoms have been there since childhood. For an adult to be diagnosed with ADHD, he/she must display at least five of the accepted symptoms. The symptoms of ADHD can change after some time, which is why adults might have different sets of symptoms compared to the ones they had when they were kids.

According to the DSM-5, ADHD presents itself in three main ways, which are – Predominantly Inattentive, Hyperactive-Impulsive, and Combined. The symptoms of each type of ADHD are as follows:

Predominantly Inattentive ADHD

- Has trouble paying close attention to details, or makes careless mistakes.

- Finds it hard to focus on just one thing.

- Always appears to not listen.

- Struggles with following basic instructions.

- Cannot keep himself/herself organized.

- Does not like to partake in tasks that require any form of sustained mental effort.

- Constantly loses or misplaces things.

- Gets distracted easily.

- Tends to be forgetful.

Hyperactive-impulsive ADHD

- Tends to fidget a lot when told to stay put in his/her chair.

- Has a hard time remaining seated.

- Always seem to be restless.

- Cannot seem to engage in activities without voicing out his/her opinions.

- Feels as if an engine is driving them about their daily lives.

- Likes to talk, a lot.

- Has difficulty letting people finish their sentences first before answering their questions.

- Dislikes waiting and abhors it when told to wait his/her turn.

- Always interrupts other people when they are talking; always interjects in other people's conversations.

Combined ADHD

This occurs when the patient meets most of the criteria for both forms of ADHD. However, these symptoms have a tendency to change after some time has passed, so the adult patients might now present different symptoms to when they were younger.

The healthcare professional will make a diagnosis of ADHD depending on the number and severity of the symptoms observed, the duration of said symptoms, and also by how much damage the symptoms have dealt to the patient's life. This means how much did the person's ADHD affect their relationships, schoolwork, or job.

As a general rule, some of the symptoms mentioned earlier must have been present before the patient turned 12 years old, which might mean that the clinician will need testimonies from the patient's parents, siblings, or anyone that is close. It is also important that there should be at least two impairments in the major settings of the patient's life. Some examples of impairments that can lead to a diagnosis of ADHD include trouble at home because of excessive conflicts, loss of a job because of not being able to concentrate on your work, getting stuck under a huge pile of debt because you always forget to pay your bills on time, and others. If the patient does not exhibit any obvious impairments, then they do not fit the criteria to be diagnosed with ADHD.

Self-diagnosis using the Internet

You can find many websites that are about ADHD, where you will find questionnaires that supposedly help you find out whether or not you have ADHD. However, these questionnaires are not standardized, nor are they validated by the medical psychiatric community and should never be used to diagnose other people with ADHD.

Who is Qualified to Diagnose ADHD?

For adults and children alike, ADHD diagnostic evaluations must only be conducted by a licensed mental health practitioner, which include clinical psychologists, physicians (psychiatrists, general practitioners, and others), and certain types of social workers.

Regardless of the type of professional you choose; it is still important to inquire about the person's educational training and experience with adults that have ADHD. Often, it is the person's experience and expertise in adult ADHD that is more important than the educational degree that they have. In any case, qualified professionals will have no problem discussing their qualifications with you.

Where Can You Find a Qualified Professional for an ADHD Diagnosis?

Now is not the time to feel ashamed to seek help if you suspect that you have ADHD; the sooner you can get diagnosed, the sooner you can get professional help to deal with this condition.

If you have a family physician, ask for a referral to a health care professional in your area who can perform ADHD diagnosis in adults.

You can also ask your insurance company for any recommendations. Usually, insurance companies provide lists of medical professionals categorized by their specialization, and you then need to choose which healthcare professional to consult. As an added bonus, the doctors listed by the insurance company's list might be covered by your existing medical plan, so you might not need to pay for a diagnosis.

How Will You Know If You Actually Need an ADHD Evaluation?

The majority of adults who undergo ADHD evaluation do so because they have experienced significant problems in one or more aspects of their personal lives. The following are the most common problems that people who have undiagnosed ADHD had to deal with:

- Inconsistent job performance, leading to stagnant careers, and/or getting fired or quitting jobs frequently

- Has a career of educational underachievement

- Has a lot of trouble managing even the most mundane daily responsibilities, such as cleaning the house, unfinished maintenance work, always late in paying the bills, and is very disorganized and messy

- Has consistent relationship problems due to the person not being able to finish tasks

- Tends to forget important events or things, and gets upset over even the most minor things

- Experiences chronic stress and worry because the patient fails to reach their goals

- Constantly feeling extreme frustration, guilt, and blames themselves

Only a qualified medical professional can determine if these problems are really caused by ADHD, by some other underlying causes, or a combination of both. Even though some symptoms of ADHD may have been evident since the patient was a child, some individuals might not notice these symptoms of ADHD until later in life. For instance, there are some smart and talented people who were able to compensate for their ADHD when they were kids and did not experience any significant problems until they reached high school, college, or until they were already a part of the workforce. In other cases, the parents of the patients sheltered them too much, thus minimizing the impact of the symptoms of ADHD during childhood.

How Should You Prepare for Your Evaluation?

Most people feel nervous and apprehensive whenever they need to get examined and evaluated for any kind of condition, and that includes ADHD testing. The stigmatization of ADHD is one of the main reasons why people do not like getting tested for it. Some of the social stigma attached to ADHD include, "It only happens to kids", and "this person is just looking for an excuse for his poor performance". As a result of this stigma, many people today are living with undiagnosed ADHD.

Many medical professionals recommend that you review your old report cards and other school records from your kindergarten and elementary school days, and better yet, bring them to your first checkup. If you previously had any psychological testing, it would also be good if you brought your records from those previous meetings as well. For adults who have trouble in the workplace, job evaluation results can also help the physician greatly to identify the source of your problem.

What Happens During a Comprehensive Examination?

Even though different clinicians will use different procedures and testing methods, there are still some protocols that are essential if you want a comprehensive evaluation of your ADHD. These protocols include a thorough diagnostic interview, information coming from independent sources like your spouse, family members, and friends, the DSM-5 symptoms checklist, and others.

Diagnostic Interview

This is the most important part of the comprehensive ADHD evaluation, and it can either be structured or semi-structured. This interview aims to provide a detailed health history of the individual. The interviewer will ask a pre-determined and standardized set of questions to the patient; these questions are designed in such a way to increase their reliability and to decrease the chances of another interviewer coming to a significantly different diagnosis. The medical professional who is conducting the interview will be covering a broad range of topics, discussing relevant subjects in as much detail as possible, and also asking follow-up questions to make sure that all possible subjects are covered. After the interview, the interviewer will then compare the results with the diagnostic criteria for ADHD to determine how many of them apply to the patient; at present, and since he/she was a child. The interviewer will also determine how much the ADHD symptoms have affected the patient's life so far.

Screening for other psychiatric disorders

The interviewer will also need to conduct another detailed review to find out if other psychiatric disorders that resemble ADHD, or co-exist with ADHD, are present. ADHD rarely manifests by itself, and scientific research has found that at least 2/3 of people who have ADHD, also have one or more underlying condition that exists alongside ADHD. The most common of these conditions includes depression, learning disabilities, and anxiety. The tricky part is that many of these conditions closely mimic the symptoms presented by ADHD, and they are often misdiagnosed as ADHD.

When the examiner discovers that the patient has one or more co-existing conditions present along with the ADHD, it is also important that those disorders are diagnosed and prescribed with adequate treatment. Failure to treat the co-existing disorders often leads to not being able to treat the ADHD as well. There are times when the ADHD is a symptom of another psychiatric disorder, like depression and anxiety. Treating the primary cause will also improve the ADHD in these cases.

The examiner will also ask about the patient's health history and that of his/her family's, academic and early work experiences, driving records and violations (if any), history of drug and alcohol abuse, family life, and others. It might seem embarrassing to pour some of this information out to the interviewer, but the information that you provide will help the examiner make a more accurate diagnosis and treatment.

Participation of loved ones

The psychiatric examiner might also require the participation of the patient's loved ones and close friends in the interview process. Usually, a person who knows the patient very well (spouse, partner, parent) is invited to answer a couple of questions. Do keep in mind that this procedure is not for confirming the honesty of the patient; this is done to gain additional information that might help. Many adults that have ADHD are not the best when it comes to remembering experiences, especially ones from their childhood. They might be able to recall a couple of specific details, but they tend to forget the problems that they experienced way back then. This is why the examiner might require the patient's parents to fill out a form that answers some questions about the person's behavior during childhood.

Another reason why the participation of the people close to the patient is necessary is because people with ADHD often have very limited awareness of how their condition is causing other people problems. For instance, in the case of married or cohabitating couples, it is best for both partners to attend the interview together. Doing so will set up the non-ADHD partner with a more accurate understanding of the other person's condition, making them more emphatic of their partner's plight; this will actually set the stage for improving the relationship.

Standardized behavior rating scales

All comprehensive evaluations include at least one standardized behavior rating scale. These are questionnaires used to compare the behavior of people with ADHD to those without the condition. Although the scores gained through the scales are not considered to be diagnostic tools by themselves, they do serve a purpose, and that is to provide objective information about the evaluation process.

Medical Examination

If the patient has not received a physical examination in the last six to twelve months, then one might be needed to rule out any medical causes for the symptoms. The examiner will not be the one to do the medical examination, the patient will most likely be referred to a duly-licensed medical physician for a proper check-up. The reason for the medical check-up is because some medical conditions have symptoms that are strikingly similar to those of ADHD, like thyroid problems.

Concluding the examination

The examiner will gather together all of the information collected through the different sources, make a written report of the findings, and then provide the patient and their family (as needed) with their diagnostic opinion about the existence of ADHD and any other conditions they believe to be present. The psychiatric examiner will then go through the available treatment options and prescribe and assist the patient with an appropriate course of action.

Chapter 3 – Common Treatments for Adult ADHD

If you are diagnosed with adult ADHD, you should not worry, it's not the end of the world. There are treatment options available that can make the condition manageable so you can continue living a regular and productive life.

Wait, There's No Cure for ADHD?

Unfortunately, there is still no known cure for Attention Deficit Hyperactivity Disorder, but there are treatments that can help the sufferer cope with the symptoms and live life as normal.

Speaking of treatments, although there are many options available, there is no one choice that can effectively minimize the effects of ADHD. Medical professionals typically advise the use of two or more treatment options in combination with each other to gain the maximum benefit.

Medications Commonly Used for ADHD

Medication may not be a permanent solution for ADHD, but they can help those who have the condition to concentrate and focus on their tasks, make them feel calm, and make them more able to learn and use new skills.

Some of these drugs must be administered every day, but some can be taken only on the weekdays when focus and concentration are most needed. Most general practitioners recommend taking treatment breaks, not only so the patient's body will not get addicted, but also to assess whether the patient still needs medication, or if they can handle the symptoms without it.

If the patient was only diagnosed with ADHD as an adult, the physician and the clinician will need to discuss suitable medication and therapy options. When you are prescribed medication, it is imperative that you let your physician know if you experience any side effects.

The ADHD specialist will discuss with you how long you should continue with your treatments, but in most cases the patients will continue treatments as long as they feel that they are helping.

There are two main types of medications that are used to treat ADHD; *stimulants* and *non-stimulants*. You will be learning about these two types, and some of the more popular examples of each type in this chapter. You will be learning about the different effects that each type of medication can have, and also the negative side effects that they have, if there are any.

Central nervous system stimulants

The most commonly prescribed class of ADHD medication are the Central Nervous System (CNS) stimulants. The way these drugs work is by increasing the brain's production of dopamine and norepinephrine, which are brain chemicals that help the brain concentrate and focus.

Some of the most common CNS stimulants that are commonly prescribed to ADHD patients include:

Amphetamine-based Stimulants

Amphetamines are stimulants that affect the chemicals in the brain; the same ones that are responsible for the person's hyperactivity and impulses. This is the reason why specialists use this to keep the symptoms of attention deficit hyperactivity disorder under control.

Aside from ADHD, certain brands, like Evekeo are also used for treating narcolepsy, and also obesity. Evekeo is commonly used by people who have tried to lose weight multiple times but have repeatedly failed.

Most amphetamines are not suitable for children who are less than 6 years old, with the exception of Evekeo, which is actually approved for use by children 3 years and older.

Important Points:

Amphetamines may be addictive, and there are many people who have abused this medication. If you have had any problems with substance abuse in the past, it is best to tell your doctor so that they can prescribe something that is less habit-forming.

Stimulants are known to cause heart attacks, strokes, and have caused sudden death in people with heart disease or who were born with a heart defect of some sort.

It is not advisable to use amphetamines if you have taken an MAO inhibitor in the last two weeks. Linezolid, phenelzine, rasagiline, selegiline, isocarboxazid, or tranylcypromine can have a bad reaction with amphetamines; the same holds true if you have received a methylene blue injection recently. Of course, your physician should have a conversation with you about any medication that you are also using before writing you a prescription.

Amphetamines might cause new, or worsen, pre-existing psychosis (unusual thoughts and strange behavior), which is especially true if you have a history of mental illness, depression, or bipolar disorder.

There is also the possibility that amphetamines might cause circulation problems, which can cause numbness and pain in your extremities.

You need to get in touch with your doctor right away if you notice: signs of heart problems, like chest pains, light-headedness, or difficulty breathing; signs of psychosis, like aggression, paranoia, hallucinations, and new behavioral problems; signs of problems with your circulation, like unexplained wounds on your fingers and toes that take a lot of time to heal.

Before you take this medication...

You must never use amphetamines if you are allergic to other kinds of stimulant medication, or if you have:

- A history of heart disease or an inborn heart defect

- High blood pressure

- An overactive thyroid gland

- Chronic anxiety as stimulants can make your symptoms worse

- A history of substance abuse; amphetamines are very habit forming, so there is a good chance that you will abuse the medication.

- Used an MAO inhibitor in the past 14 days, as there could be a dangerous interaction between the amphetamine and the inhibitor

Some medications have been discovered to have a negative interaction with amphetamines and have caused a serious medical condition known as serotonin syndrome, which is characterized by high fever, diarrhea, and other symptoms. If left untreated serotonin syndrome could cause seizures and rapid and extensive muscle breakdown.

You need to let your doctor know if you are taking other medications like opioids, herbal products, or medication for depression, Parkinson's, other mental illnesses, chronic migraines, antibiotics, and others. You need to ask your doctor before you make any change in your medications, and the time that you take them.

To ensure that you can safely use amphetamines, you need to tell your doctor if you, or anyone in your family has ever had:

- Depression, bipolar disorder, psychosis, or any other mental illness

- Harbored suicidal thoughts, or displayed suicidal tendencies

- Problems regarding substance abuse

- Facial tics or Tourette's syndrome

- Kidney diseases

- Thyroid disorders

- Epilepsy or prone to seizures

- An unusual brain wave test (EEG)

- Clogged arteries

- Circulation problems in the hands and/or the feet

You should also tell your attending physician if you are an expecting a baby. Taking this medication during pregnancy can cause premature birth, cause the baby to be born undersized, or the withdrawal symptoms could arise in the baby as well. You need to tell your doctor if you are pregnant, or if you are planning to get pregnant in the near future so that you can get a prescription for another type of medication.

Amphetamines can also pass into breastmilk and may cause harm to a nursing baby. You need to tell your doctor if you are breastfeeding a child so that you can get an alternative prescription.

How to Take Amphetamines

If you use amphetamines haphazardly, it could cause serious addiction, damage the heart, or even cause death.

You need to follow all the directions as prescribed by your doctor or as written on the instruction sheets.

Amphetamines are habit-forming, so you should never share your prescription amphetamines with others, especially with someone who has had a history of substance abuse and addiction. Also remember that selling, or even giving away, some of your meds to other people is illegal and could land you in prison.

You can take amphetamines with or without eating first, and they should always be taken in the morning. If you take amphetamines too late in the day, like in the early evening, you might find it hard to sleep.

If ever your physician changes the brand or strength of your stimulant medicine, the amount you need to take might change as well. You need to use the brand and strength that your doctor has specified to avoid complications.

If you are using an oral liquid form of medication, you should shake the container well before you measure a dose. You should always measure the amount of liquid medication with the dosing cup or syringe included in the packaging.

If you are going to take orally soluble tablets:

Let the tablets remain in their blister packs until you are ready to take them. When you are ready to take your pills, using clean, dry hands, peel away the protective foil. You should not push the tablet through popping the foil as it might damage the tablet.

Use a dry hand to pop the pill into your mouth.

Do not swallow the tablet. Allow it to rest on top of your tongue and let it dissolve without chewing. If you want, you can sip a bit of water to help yourself swallow the tablet.

When you are using amphetamines, your doctor will be checking on you from time to time to see your progress. You need to tell all doctors that you are seeing that you are taking amphetamines for your ADHD so they will not prescribe medications that will cause a negative reaction.

What if I miss a dose?

As soon as you remember that you missed a dose, take it immediately if it's not too late in the day. Do not take a double dose the following day, as this will only increase the chances of developing an addiction.

What will happen if I overdose?

You need to seek emergency medical attention. Overdosing on amphetamines can be fatal.

When you overdose on amphetamines, here are some of the symptoms that might arise: muscle pain or weakness, dark-colored urine, muscle twitching, unexplained hostility, thoughts of violence, and others. In some of the worst cases, overdosing might also cause seizures or put you in a coma.

Things I need to avoid while I am taking amphetamines:

While you are taking amphetamines to take care of your ADHD, you need to avoid drinking alcoholic beverages.

You should also avoid drinking fruit juices, and stop taking vitamin C as it will make your body less able to absorb the medication.

Do not drive, operate heavy machinery, or do any sort of hazardous activity until you know for sure what kind of effect the amphetamine will have on you. There is a chance that your reaction time could be impaired, so be careful when first taking the medication.

Side Effects of Amphetamines

If you are showing signs of a severe allergic reaction to the medication, like breaking out in hives, have difficulty breathing, swelling of the face, tongue, or throat, and others, then you need to call 911 and get immediate medical help.

You need to call your doctor when you:

- See signs of heart problems - chest pain, difficulty breathing, lightheadedness, and others.

- See signs of psychosis – hallucinations, unexplained aggression, paranoia, sudden hostility, and new behavioral problems that were not there before.

- See signs of circulation problems – when you feel sudden numbness and coldness in your fingers and toes, or if the skin in your extremities suddenly changes color (gets pale, reddens, or gets blue). Also, when you suddenly get small wounds in your fingertips for unexplained reasons.

- Experience a seizure

- Suddenly develop muscle twitches

- Suddenly get blurry vision

You will need immediate medical attention if you start to notice the symptoms of serotonin syndrome, such as:

- Getting easily agitated

- Suddenly experiencing hallucinations

- Have a high fever for several days

- Excessive sweating

- Uncontrollable shivering

- Raised heart rate

- Muscle stiffness

- Sudden loss of coordination

- Nausea and vomiting

- Diarrhea

Common Side Effects of Amphetamines:

- Cottonmouth

- An unusual/unpleasant taste in the mouth

- Sudden loss of appetite

- Sudden weight loss

- Stomach pain and diarrhea

- Constantly feeling restless or full of nerves

- Insomnia

- Sudden mood swings

- Dizziness, nausea, and a slight fever

Dextromethamphetamine (Desoxyn)

Dextroamphetamine, also known as d-amphetamine, just like amphetamines, is a stimulant that somewhat enhances the performance of the central nervous system. This drug increases the production of brain chemicals and stimulates the nerves that contribute to hyperactivity and impulsivity. Aside from ADHD, dextroamphetamine is also used to treat narcolepsy and other sleep disorders.

Important Points:

You should not use d-amphetamine if you are suffering from glaucoma, hyperthyroidism, severe agitation, high blood pressure and other heart diseases, or if you have a history of substance abuse.

D-amphetamine is highly addictive, and there are many cases of people abusing this drug. This is why you need to tell your ADHD examiner if you have a history of drug and alcohol abuse so they can prescribe another treatment option that is less hazardous for you.

Stimulants like d-amphetamine have caused strokes, heart attacks, and sudden death in people who have heart diseases or inborn heart defects.

You should not use d-amphetamine if you used an MAO inhibitor in the past 2 weeks. MAO inhibitors include isocarboxazid, linezolid, methylene blue injection, phenelzine, rasagiline, selegiline, or tranylcypromine.

D-amphetamine can also cause new cases of or worsen existing psychosis. This is especially true if you have a history of mental illness or depression.

Use of stimulants like d-amphetamine can also cause circulation problems which can then cause numbness, slight pain, and discoloration of the skin in your extremities.

You need to call your doctor right away if you experience the following after taking d-amphetamine: chest pain, light headedness, shortness of breath; early signs of psychosis, like paranoia, unexplained aggression, sudden changes in behavior, and hallucinations; signs of circulation problems, like numb/tingly sensation in the fingers and toes.

Before you take d-amphetamine

You should never use d-amphetamine if you are found to be allergic to stimulant medication, or if you have:

- High blood pressure or any other heart disease

- Hyperthyroidism

- Chronic anxiety, tension, or are easily agitated; stimulants will make all of these conditions much worse

- A history of substance abuse, or if you are a recovering drug addict or alcoholic

You should never use d-amphetamine if you have used an MAO inhibitor in the last 2 weeks, or else it will result in a very dangerous interaction between the two medications.

Just like amphetamines, certain types of medication can also interact negatively with d-amphetamine to cause a very dangerous health condition called serotonin syndrome. You need to tell your ADHD examiner if you are currently taking other types of medication such as, opioids, herbal remedies, or if you are also taking medication for mental illnesses, Parkinson's, or if you are taking antibiotics to counter a serious infection. You should consult with your doctor first before making any changes to your other medications.

There are many reports of stimulant medication that has caused fatal strokes and heart attacks. This is why you need to tell your doctor if you have:

- Heart disease or a congenital heart defect

- High blood pressure, or if you have a family history of having heart conditions.

To ensure that it is safe for you to take d-amphetamine, you need to tell your physician if anyone in your family has:

- Depression, bipolar disorder, psychosis, or if you have had suicidal thoughts

- Facial tics, or Tourette's syndrome

- Epilepsy or seizures

- Abnormal brainwave test results

- Circulation problems, mainly in the extremities

Just like with amphetamines, taking d-amphetamine during pregnancy could cause miscarriages, premature birth, very low birth weight, or cause the baby to suffer from withdrawal symptoms. You really should tell your physician and your ADHD examiner if you are pregnant, or if you plan to be in the near future so they can prescribe other forms of treatment that will not put the baby at risk.

D-amphetamine can also pass through the mother's breastmilk, which might harm a nursing baby. You should find other forms of medication if you are currently nursing a child.

D-amphetamine is not approved for use by children 3 years old and below. The extended release d-amphetamine capsules on the other hand are not approved for use by children aged 6 and below.

How to take d-amphetamine?

You need to strictly follow the instructions on your prescription. Your attending physician might occasionally change the size of the dosages, depending on how well you have been coping. Do not take dextroamphetamine in bigger or smaller amounts without the knowledge of your doctor.

The standard dosage of d-amphetamine is usually 2-3 times a day, or as needed. There is also extended-release d-amphetamine, where one tablet can last an entire day. However, your dosage may vary, so follow what your doctor orders.

Speaking of extended-release d-amphetamine, you should never chew, crush, or open up an extended-release capsule. You need to swallow it whole. The casing of the capsule will be responsible for the timed release of the contents.

D-amphetamine is a habit-forming drug. You should never share your medication with someone else. You need to keep this and all of your other medication somewhere where other people can't get to it. And remember, selling or giving away of d-amphetamine is punishable by law.

Your doctor will need to check up on your progress regularly, so you need to be honest with them if you have been able to follow the prescribed dosage so far, and if you are experiencing any negative side effects as a result of your medication.

What if you miss a dose?

Take the missed dose immediately when you remember, however, if it is already the early evening or later then just skip it. If you take a stimulant this late in the day, you will find it very difficult to sleep later. You should never take a double dosage of d-amphetamine to make up for your missed dose, it does not work this way, and doing so will only increase your risk of addiction.

What to do when you overdose?

Overdosing on d-amphetamine can be very dangerous. You need to call emergency medical services or the Poison Help line (1-800-222-1222).

The symptoms of overdosing on d-amphetamine include:

- Restlessness

- The shakes

- Muscles twitching

- Confusion

- Hallucinations

- Sudden aggressive behavior

- Lightheadedness

- Seizures

- Fainting spells

Things to avoid while taking d-amphetamine

D-amphetamine can cloud your judgment and impair your reaction time. It is advisable that you do not drive or operate any heavy machinery while you are taking d-amphetamine.

Do not consume any fruit juices or vitamin C supplements when you are taking d-amphetamine. Vitamin C makes your body absorb less of the d-amphetamine.

Side effects of d-amphetamine

You need to seek emergency medical services the moment that you see signs of an allergic reaction to d-amphetamine. Here are some of the signs that you need to keep an eye out for:

- Breaking out in hives

- Difficulty breathing

- Swelling in the face, tongue, and throat

You also need to call your doctor if you experience:

- Signs of heart problems, like chest pains, difficulty breathing, lightheadedness, etc.

- Signs of psychosis, like hallucinations, new behavioral problems, trouble controlling your aggression, and paranoia.

- Signs of circulation problems, like numbness/tingling sensations in your fingers and toes, and unexplained small wounds that take a long time to heal completely.

- Seizures

- Facial tics

- Sudden changes in your vision

You should also seek medical attention when you start displaying the symptoms associated with serotonin syndrome, such as:

- Easily getting agitated

- Hallucinations

- High fever that comes and goes

- Sweats a lot, even when you just came out of the shower

- Uncontrollable shaking

- Increased heart rate

- Sudden loss of coordination

- Nausea, vomiting, and/or diarrhea

Common side effects of d-amphetamine include, but are not limited to:

- Cottonmouth

- Upset stomach

- Sudden loss of appetite and unhealthy weight loss

- Chronic headaches, sudden dizziness spells

- Hand tremors, increased heart rate

- Insomnia

Dextromethylphenidate (Focalin)

Unlike the first two medications discussed, dextromethylphenidate, also called dexmethylphenidate, is a mild stimulant for the central nervous system. However, just like amphetamine and d-amphetamine, dexmethylphenidate also affects the production of the brain chemicals that are responsible for regulating hyperactivity and impulse control.

Important Points

You should not use stimulants like dexmethylphenidate if you are suffering from glaucoma, Tourette's syndrome, tension, severe anxiety, or if you are easily agitated. Taking stimulants with these condition will only worsen your symptoms.

Although dexmethylphenidate is a milder stimulant compared to amphetamines, it is still habit-forming. You should tell your doctor and your ADHD examiner if you have a history of substance abuse, so you can get prescribed another type of medication that will not risk addiction.

Stimulants, even mild ones, have been known to cause strokes, heart attacks, and even sudden death in people who have congenital heart defects/diseases.

There is also a distinct possibility that dexmethylphenidate can cause new, or worsen existing psychosis. This is especially true when you have a history of mental illnesses, bipolar disorder, depression, and other mental illnesses.

You might also experience blood circulation problems, particularly in your extremities, like your fingers and toes. You might feel a bit of pain, numbness or tingling, or discoloration of the skin.

Before you take dexmethylphenidate

You should not take this if you are highly allergic to dexmethylphenidate or methylphenidate (Ritalin, Concerta), or if you have:

- Glaucoma

- Tourette's syndrome, or if anyone in your family has it

- Extreme anxiety, tension, or if you are easily agitated; taking stimulants will make these symptoms much worse.

You must not use dexmethylphenidate of you took an MAO inhibitor in the past two weeks as a dangerous interaction between the two might occur. MAO inhibitors include, but are not limited to the following:

- isocarboxazid

- linezolid

- methylene blue injection

- phenelzine

- rasagiline

- selegiline

- tranylcypromine

Certain medicines might interact differently with dexmethylphenidate and cause a serious health condition known as serotonin syndrome. You need to let your doctor and your ADHD examiner know if:

- You are taking opioid medicines

- Herbal products

- Medication for depression, Parkinson's, and other mental illnesses

- Antibiotics for serious infections

- Medication against nausea and vomiting

You should not decide on your own to stop using your other medications just so you can use dexmethylphenidate. You need to ask your doctor before making changes in your medication dosage and schedule.

Even mild CNS stimulants like dexmethylphenidate have caused strokes, heart attacks, and unexplained and sudden death in certain individuals who have heart disease and/or congenital heart defects.

You need to inform your doctor if you have:

- A congenital heart defect or other kinds of heart problems

- High blood pressure

- A family with a history of heart disease and stroke

In addition, you need to ensure that your doctor knows if you or anyone in your family has ever had:

- Depression, bipolar disorder, psychosis, or have harbored suicidal thoughts and tendencies

- Involuntary motor tics, or Tourette's syndrome

- Blood circulation problems, particularly in the extremities

- Epileptic episodes or seizures

- Abnormal brain wave test results

- Problems with addiction

Just like the other stimulants, dexmethylphenidate is not advisable for use by pregnant or breastfeeding women. Use of dexmethylphenidate while pregnant can induce premature birth, cause the baby to have a very low birth weight, or the baby might experience withdrawal symptoms. You need to inform your doctor and your ADHD examiner if you are pregnant or if you are planning to get pregnant, so you can get a different treatment program that does not include stimulants.

It is still unclear whether dexmethylphenidate can pass through the breastmilk of mothers, and if it does, if it will harm the nursing baby. However, just to be sure, you should consult with your doctor first before going through with the treatment while breastfeeding.

How to take dexmethylphenidate

Even though this is just a mild stimulant, it is still important that you follow the prescription label when taking dexmethylphenidate. There will be times when your doctor will make adjustments to your dosages, and that is fine. Deciding on your own that you need more or less of the medication is not something you should do.

You need to read and understand all of the patient information, guides, and instructions provided to you by your doctor. If you have any questions or you want to clarify anything, just ask your doctor.

Keep in mind that dexmethylphenidate might be addictive. This is why you should never share your prescription medications with anyone else.

Dexmethylphenidate can be taken on an empty stomach. The regular tablet should be taken twice a day, with at least four hours in between dosages. If you are taking the extended-release capsules, you only need to take one a day; early in the morning is recommended. However, it is unadvisable to take it late in the afternoon as it might make it difficult to sleep.

Never chew, crush, or open up an extended-release capsule. These are intended to be swallowed whole; the casing will take care of releasing the right amount of the medication over time.

Your doctor will be closely monitoring you once you start using dexmethylphenidate. During every visit to the clinic, your doctor will likely check your heart rate, blood pressure, and other vitals just to make sure that nothing is out of sync.

What to do when you miss a dose?

You need to take the missed dose as soon as you are reminded of it, but not if it is already late in the day. If it's late in the day, just remember to take your dose the next day and avoid double-dosing.

What to do if you overdose?

You need to seek emergency medical care as soon as you notice that you might have overdosed on your medication. Either call 911 or the Poison Help line (1-800-222-1222).

The symptoms that you might encounter when you overdose on dexmethylphenidate include:

- Sudden restlessness

- Hand tremors

- Facial muscles begin twitching

- Rapid shallow breathing

- Confusion and panic

- Hallucinations

- Muscle pain or weakness

- Dark-colored urine

If you really went overboard with the dosage, the following symptoms will arise, and by this stage you definitely need emergency medical attention:

- Nausea

- Vomiting

- Diarrhea

- Irregular heartbeat

- Lightheadedness and fainting

- Seizures

- Unconsciousness

Things to avoid while taking dexmethylphenidate

You need to avoid taking dexmethylphenidate in the late afternoon or early in the evening as it might cause you to experience sleep problems, namely insomnia.

Dexmethylphenidate can cause blurry vision and dull your reaction time. See how you react to the medication first before driving a vehicle.

Side effects of dexmethylphenidate

As always, you need to get immediate medical help if you see the signs of an allergic reaction, like hives, or a high fever. If you ignore the symptoms and it gets worse, which can happen quickly, then next symptoms may be the swelling of your face, tongue, and even your throat, thus preventing you from breathing.

The following symptoms also require medical attention if they are experienced:

- Signs of heart problems, like chest pains, difficulty breathing, lightheadedness, and feeling like you might faint.

- Signs of psychosis, like hallucinations, sudden new behavioral patterns, aggressive behavior and hostility, bouts of paranoia, and others.

- Signs of circulation problems, like numbness and tingling of the fingers and toes, sudden unexplained wounds in the fingers, and the skin of the extremities also changes color to red, and sometimes even blue.

- Minor to moderate seizures

- Blurry vision

- For males, a painful erection that lasts for four hours, or
  longer.

Aside from the side effects from the dexmethylphenidate, you
should also watch out for the effects of serotonin syndrome,
which sometimes happens when two different medications
affect each other. Here are the symptoms:

- Hallucinations

- Moderate to high fever

- Excessive sweating

- Shivering

- Increased heart rate

- Pain and stiffness in the muscles

- Nervous tic

- Loss of coordination

- Nausea

- Vomiting

- Diarrhea

Common side effects of dexmethylphenidate

- Sudden loss of appetite

- Nausea

- Moderate fever

Methylphenidate (Concerta, Daytrana, Metadate, Ritalin)

Just like the other stimulants in this list, methylphenidate is a stimulant that acts upon the central nervous system. This medication affects the production of certain brain chemicals; the ones that contribute to hyperactivity and impulsivity, which are some of the most common symptoms of ADHD.

Aside from ADHD, methylphenidate can also treat narcolepsy.

Important points to consider

Methylphenidate, just like most other stimulants, might be habit-forming, and there are numerous cases of people abusing this prescription medication. You need to inform your physician and your ADHD examiner if you have a history of substance abuse.

There have been numerous reports of stimulants causing strokes, heart attacks, and sudden death in people who have high blood pressure or have a history of heart disease.

You should avoid using methylphenidate if you used an MAO inhibitor in the last two weeks.

Methylephenidate might cause psychosis in certain individuals, which is the emergence of strange, foreboding thoughts in the mind of the sufferer. If the person already has some form of psychosis already, taking methylphenidate might worsen its symptoms.

The medication might cause slight blood circulation problems, which can cause numbness, pain, or a tingling sensation in the fingers and/or toes. The finger tips and tips of the toes might even have a bit of discoloration. Sometimes, cuts or bruises on your hands and/or feet may appear.

Before taking methylphenidate

First of all, you need to determine if you are allergic to methylphenidate, and if you are you need to inform your physician about it. You should also not use methylphenidate if you have:

- Glaucoma

- A family history of Tourette's syndrome, severe anxiety, tension, and similar conditions. Taking stimulants like methylphenidate will only make the symptoms of these conditions much worse.

- Recently had a heart attack.

- Severe hypertension, experienced heart failure, have an irregular heartbeat, or other heart diseases.

- Hyperthyroidism

Since stimulants have caused quite a number of fatal strokes, heart attacks, and sometimes even sudden death in people who have weak hearts, it is important to tell your doctor if you have:

- Heart problems or a congenital heart disease

- High blood pressure

- A family history of high blood pressure and sudden death due to heart attacks and strokes

To ensure that it is safe for you to use methylphenidate, you need to inform your doctor if you or anyone in your immediate family has ever had:

- A history of mental illnesses such as depression, bipolar disorder, psychosis, or if you have ever had suicidal thoughts or tendencies.

- Facial twitch due to stress

- Problems with blood circulation

- Recent bouts with epileptic seizures

- Gastrointestinal problems

- Problems with alcohol or drug addiction

It is still unclear if methylphenidate has any harmful effects on unborn babies. But just to be sure, you should tell your physician before you are prescribed with an ADHD treatment program if you are pregnant, or if you are planning to get pregnant in the near future.

It is also not known if methylphenidate can get into a mother's breastmilk or if it could harm a breastfeeding baby. Either way, it is important to tell your doctor if you are breastfeeding.

If you will need to undergo surgery, you need to tell your surgeon that you are taking methylphenidate. You should also tell your doctor that you will be undergoing surgery, regardless if it is minor or major surgery. You might need to stop taking methylphenidate for a while, or your doctor might prescribe another form of medication for the meantime.

How to take methylphenidate?

You should follow your doctor's prescription to the letter. Do not add or subtract from the amount prescribed by your physician; your doctor will make adjustments for you occasionally when they notice that you need either more or if you can do with less.

Methylphenidate could be addictive, so you should never share your prescription medications with another person, especially if said person has a history of drug abuse. You should keep your medications in a safe place that only you have access to.

Also keep in mind that selling and even giving away your ADHD medications, especially the amphetamines and other stimulants, is against the law and might land you in jail.

As with all stimulants, as much as possible, methylphenidate should be taken in the morning, especially the extended-release capsules. Taking them during the afternoon or early evening will cause sleep problems.

The regular methylphenidate should be placed under your tongue and allowed to dissolve in your mouth. However, the extended-release methylphenidate should be swallowed whole; you must not chew, crush, or open the capsule.

What should I do if I miss a dose?

Take the dose as soon as you are reminded of it. However, if it is already late in the afternoon, or later than 6PM, just let the missed dose slide. Taking it late in the day might make it difficult for you to sleep come bedtime. Do not take a double dose the next day to compensate.

What to do if I overdose?

Overdosing on methylphenidate might be fatal so you need to call 911 immediately, or you can call the Poison Help Line hotline at 1-800-222-1222. Do this as soon as you realize that you might have taken a larger dose than you are supposed to.

What to avoid while you are taking methylphenidate?

You need to stop drinking alcohol, especially when you are taking the extended-release methylphenidate. The alcohol in your beverages will cause the medication to be released into your bloodstream way too fast.

You should also avoid driving or operating heavy machinery until you know how your body reacts to the methylphenidate. If you feel fine after a week or so of continued use of methylphenidate, then you can drive and operate heavy machines again.

Side effects of methylphenidate

If you see the early signs of an allergic reaction to methylphenidate, like hives or slight difficulty breathing, then you need to take yourself to the emergency room right away. If it gets worse, such as swelling of your face, mouth and tongue, you need to call an ambulance.

You need to call your doctor immediately if you have:

- Signs of heart problems like, acute chest pain, difficulty breathing, lightheadedness, and constantly feeling faint.

- Signs of psychosis, like hallucinations, sudden changes in behavior, quick to anger, hostile to everything and everyone, and paranoia.

- Signs of problems with blood circulation, like when you suddenly feel numbness, tingling, unexplained wounds suddenly appearing on your fingers and toes.

- Sudden seizures or epileptic episodes.

- Twitching facial muscles when stressed.

- Sudden blurring of your vision.

- For males, a painful erection that lasts four hours or more.

Common side effects of methylphenidate

- Sudden mood changes

- Always feeling nervous

- Always irritable

- Trouble sleeping (insomnia)

- Increased heart rate

- Increased blood pressure

- Sudden weight loss, loss of appetite

- Nausea

- Stomach pains

- Constant migraines

Nonstimulant Medications

Your doctor might consider switching you over to nonstimulant medication if the stimulants did not work for you, or if the side effects are too much for you to handle.

Certain nonstimulant medications help by increasing the levels of norepinephrine in your brain. This substance is said to help with improving attention and memory.

There are many nonstimulant treatments available, and here are some of the most popular:

Atomoxetine

Atomoxetine tweaks the levels of brain chemicals and the nerves that play huge roles in hyperactivity and impulsivity.

Important Points

You must not use atomoxetine if you are suffering from glaucoma, a tumor in your adrenal gland, heart disease, or high blood pressure.

Just like with stimulants, you should not use atomoxetine if you have taken an MAO inhibitor in the last two weeks; the combination of these two medications might result in a dangerous adverse reaction.

Atomoxetine may also cause psychosis in the user, or if the user already has a pre-existing psychosis, taking this medication can make the symptoms even worse. This is especially true if you are suffering from depression, severe mental illness, or if you have bipolar disorder.

There are plenty of reports of atomoxetine inducing strokes, heart attacks, and even sudden death in people who are also suffering from heart disease, or have a congenital heart defect.

Some people report having had suicidal thoughts the first time they took atomoxetine, or when their dosage was changed. You need to pay close attention to any changes in your mood, especially if you had suicidal tendencies in the past.

Before using atomoxetine

You need to stop using atomoxetine if you are allergic to it, or if you:

- Have a severe heart disease or if there are problems with your blood vessels

- Have glaucoma

Atomoxetine has caused certain people to have heart attacks and strokes, which is why you need to tell your doctor if you have:

- Heart disease, or if you have a congenital heart defect

- Moderate to severe blood pressure

- A family history of heart disease and stroke

- Mental illnesses, like depression, bipolar disorder, and psychosis

- Suicidal thoughts, or if anyone in your family has ever committed suicide

- Extremely low blood pressure

- Liver disease

It is important that when you go to your doctor for your regular check-ups, you to tell your doctor about any suicidal thoughts you may have had, so that an appropriate change to your dosage can be made.

It is still unknown whether or not atomoxetine has any effects on unborn babies. It is best to tell your doctor immediately if you are pregnant, or if you have plans to become pregnant.

It is also not yet confirmed whether or not atomoxetine can pass from the bloodstream and into breastmilk. Just to be on the safe side, you should tell your doctor if you are breastfeeding.

How to take atomoxetine

You need to follow all the instructions on your prescription label. Always read the label because your doctor might occasionally change the dosage in your prescription from time to time. Never take atomoxetine in a larger or smaller amount than what your doctor has prescribed.

Take atomoxetine at the same time every day, and with a glass of water. The usual prescriptions of atomoxetine are once-a-day (often early in the morning) and two-times-a-day (once in the morning and another for the afternoon).

Atomoxetine can be taken with or without sustenance.

When taking atomoxetine, you should not crush, chew, or break open the atomoxetine capsule. You need to swallow it whole.

To get the greatest benefit, you need to use atomoxetine regularly according to your prescription, without missing days if possible. This is why it is also important to get your prescription medication refilled before your bottle is empty.

Your doctor will be continuously monitoring your progress during your regular clinic visits. They will likely check your heart rate, blood pressure, and other vital statistics. If any of them seem irregular, your doctor will adjust your dosage or completely replace your medication with an alternative.

What to do if you miss a dose

It is important that you take the dose immediately when you remember it. However, you should just skip the dose altogether if it is late in the day.

Do not double your dosage to make up for the skipped dosage earlier.

What to do if you overdose

You need to seek emergency medical treatment by calling 911, or you could call the Poison Help line at 1-800-222-1222.

What should you avoid while taking atomoxetine?

Avoid using or handling a broken capsule. If the powdered medication contained inside the capsule ever gets into your eyes, it can cause severe irritation. Rinse your eyes thoroughly with clean water and call your doctor in this case.

There is a chance that atomoxetine will impair your judgment and slow down your reflexes, which is a dangerous combination to have when you are behind the wheel of a motorized vehicle. It is recommended that you do not drive or operate any heavy machinery until you know exactly how your body will react to atomoxetine. Leave the driving to someone else for a week or so, or until your body gets used to the medication.

Common side effects of atomoxetine

The moment that you notice the signs of a severe allergic reaction, like breaking out in hives or having slight difficulty breathing, then you need to call your doctor. However, if your face, tongue, and mouth begin swelling up fast, you need to get to the emergency room as quickly as you can.

You should also inform your doctor if you notice any new or worsening symptoms, like panic attacks, sleep problems, or increased anxiety, or if you start to feel impulsive, always irritable, hostile and aggressive towards the people around you, restless, or depressed. Call your doctor or a suicide prevention hotline if you start to have suicidal thoughts or if you are thinking of hurting yourself.

Call your doctor if you suddenly have:

- Signs of heart problems, like chest pains, trouble breathing, or if you feel like you might pass out at any time.

- Signs of psychosis, like experiencing hallucinations, sudden changes in your behavior, extreme aggressiveness and hostility towards other people, and paranoia.

- Liver problems; when you start feeling abdominal pain (upper right side of your tummy), flu-like symptoms, dark-colored urine, and jaundice (yellowing of the skin and eyes).

- Painful urination

- (if you are a man) a painful erection that often lasts four hours or more.

- Cottonmouth

- Loss of appetite

- Violent mood swings

- Constantly drained of energy

- Always nauseated

- Upset stomach and constipation

Antidepressants like nortriptyline (Pamelor)

Nortriptyline is a kind of tricyclic antidepressant, which means it affects the levels of brain chemicals that might be unbalanced in people who are suffering from depression. This effect of nortriptyline is also one of the reasons why it is used to treat ADHD as well.

Important points

It is important that you do not use nortriptyline if you recently just had a heart attack, or if you have allergic reactions to several types of medication

Do not use nortriptyline if you used an MAO inhibitor in the last 14 days.

Some patients have reported suicidal thoughts and intentions upon first taking antidepressants. This is the reason why your doctor needs to monitor you closely while you are on nortriptyline. Your doctor should also inform your family or caregivers to keep an eye out for any sudden mood changes that you might not be aware of.

If you do find any worsening symptoms, like changes in your mood and usual behavior, such as trouble sleeping, panic attacks, extreme anxiety, or irritability, then contact your doctor.

Before taking nortriptyline

Immediately stop using nortriptyline if you experience the early signs of an allergic reaction after taking the medication for the first time. The early signs would be itchiness and redness of the skin. When you see these signs, go directly to the emergency rooms so you can get first aid.

You should not use nortriptyline if you recently just suffered from a heart attack.

If you are allergic to certain antidepressant medications like amoxapine, doxepin, protriptyline, and others, then you might be allergic to nortriptyline as well. The same goes if you are allergic to certain seizure meds like carbamazepine and rufinamide.

To ensure that nortriptyline is safe for you to use, you need to tell your doctor of you have:

- Any kind of heart disease, or if you have a history of heart attack, stroke, or epileptic seizures

- Bipolar disorder, schizophrenia, and other mental disorders

- Liver disease

- Hyperthyroidism or hypothyroidism

- Diabetes

- Glaucoma

- Urinary tract infection, or if you have trouble urinating lately

- Pregnant, planning to get pregnant, or if you are a nursing mother

Suicidal thoughts have been reported when first taking nortriptyline. If you experience this side effect then contact your doctor immediately so that they can make the necessary changes to your dosage, or prescribe you a different medication altogether.

How to take nortriptyline?

You should always follow the dosage as prescribed by your physician. Do not change your dosage without first contacting your doctor.

If you will be undergoing surgery, tell the surgeon in advance that you are currently taking nortriptyline. In some cases, you may need to stop taking nortriptyline for a while.

You should not suddenly stop taking nortriptyline or else you may experience unpleasant withdrawal symptoms. If you feel that you need to stop using this medication, ask your doctor for the safest way to quit.

Do not expect your ADHD symptoms to improve the moment you first take nortriptyline; it might take a couple of weeks before you can start seeing noticeable improvements. If a couple of weeks have already passed and you still feel like nothing has happened, then you need to consult with your doctor.

What to do if you miss a dose?

You need to take the dose as soon as you remember, unless it is already late in the day. It is also important to remember that you should not take an extra dose to make up for the one you missed.

What happens if you overdose?

If you take too much nortriptyline, the you may begin to feel chest pain, lightheadedness, drowsiness, and begin vomiting. If this happens, you need to call for emergency medical attention, or you could call the Poison Help line (1-800-222-1222). You should do this immediately because overdosing on nortriptyline can be fatal.

Things to avoid while you are on nortriptyline

You should quit drinking alcoholic beverages. Nortriptyline can actually increase the effects of alcohol, which might sound fun, but it is actually dangerous because it increases your chances of succumbing to alcohol poisoning.

Nortriptyline can impair your reaction time and cloud your judgment. You might want to hold off on driving your car to work or operate any kind of heavy machinery for a week or so until you know exactly how nortriptyline will affect you.

Avoid standing under the sun for an extended period. Taking nortriptyline can actually make you more prone to sunburn.

You need to regularly use sunscreen (at least SPF 30 or higher) to prevent your skin from getting burned.

When to seek medical attention

You need to get immediate medical assistance if you notice the signs of allergic reaction, like your skin breaking out in hives, or if your face, lips, or tongue starts to swell up.

You should also report to your doctor if you have experienced any new or worsened symptoms, like if you suddenly became easily irritable, hostile and aggressive to the people around you. You also need to report if any of your existing symptoms actually got worse, like you have gotten even more depressed than before, and you have started contemplating suicide or self-harm.

You should also immediately call your doctor if you experienced blurry vision, tunnel vision (when the edges of your field of vision suddenly get blurry), eye pain, or if you are starting to see halos around lights.

Other symptoms that you need to tell your doctor about include:

- Muscle twitching in your eyes, jaw, tongue, or in your neck

- Feeling lightheaded, like you are constantly feeling like fainting

- Epileptic seizures

- Increased heart rate and chest pains

- Sudden numbness or weakness in the extremities, problems with your vision, slurred speech, or sudden loss of balance

- High fever that lasts a couple of days

- Bruising easily

- Jaundice (yellowish skin and eyes)

- Painful urination

- Hallucinations

There are other, less-popular nonstimulant drugs that can also help keep the symptoms of ADHD at bay. However, it is not fully known how the following medications actually help, but there is some evidence showing that they improve the levels of brain chemicals that are in charge of attention and memory.

These other non-stimulant medications include:

Guanfacine (Intuniv)

Guanfacine works by reducing the amount of nerve impulses in the heart and blood vessels. This drug relaxes the blood vessels, which in turn lowers blood pressure and improves the flow of blood.

The Tenex brand of guanfacine is the one commonly used to treat hypertension, and it is sometimes taken with other kinds of high blood pressure medications. The Intuniv brand on the other hand is used for treating ADHD in adults.

Important Points

You need to follow the directions on your doctor's prescription. You also need to tell all of your doctors (dentists, dermatologists, general practice, etc.) about your medical condition and the medications that you are currently using.

Before taking guanfacine

You should first make sure that you are not allergic to guanfacine before you use it. Generally, your doctor will do a test patch on your skin to find out if you are allergic to the medication or not.

In addition, you should tell your doctor if you have a history of:

- Heart diseases like coronary artery disease (clogged arteries)

- Irregular heartbeat

- Heart attack or stroke

- Moderate to severe high blood pressure

- Moderate to severe low blood pressure

- Liver ailments

- Kidney ailments

How to take guanfacine?

You need to follow your doctor's directions on the prescription, and you should also read the medication guides or the instructions on the label of the medication.

You should not modify your dosage in any way; do not take more or less than what your doctor prescribed. Your doctor might change your dosage occasionally if your condition gets better.

You should take Intuniv with a glass of water, milk, or any other liquid you like.

You need to swallow the Intuniv tablet whole; do not chew, crush, or break the capsule.

Do not stop using guanfacine all of a sudden. Doing so will raise your blood pressure and cause unpleasant withdrawal symptoms. You need to talk with your doctor if you want to stop using guanfacine for any reason. Your doctor will advise you on the best course of action to take, and maybe even give you an alternative medication option that has milder side effects.

If your doctor switches you to a different brand, strength, or form of guanfacine, then the amount of your dosages will need to change as well. You can avoid committing medication errors if you just use the form and strength as prescribed by your doctor.

Your doctor will need to check your progress regularly to see if your medications are having the desired effect. You will likely need to visit the clinic at least once a month, or your doctor might task you with measuring your own blood pressure and heart rate daily from home, and then send your results to them via email.

What do I do if I miss a dose?

You should avoid taking guanfacine after eating high-fat foods as this will cause your body to absorb the medicine faster than anticipated.

If you forgot a dose, take it as soon as you remember. However, skip it altogether if it is almost time for your next dosage. You should not take two doses at one time, nor should you take two doses within an hour of each other.

What to do if you overdose?

When you notice the first symptoms of overdosing on medication, you need to get to the emergency room as quick as possible, or you can call the Poison Help line (1-800-222-1222).

The symptoms of overdosing can include, but are not limited to:

- Drowsiness

- Very slow heart rate

- Feeling like you will pass out at any minute

Things you need to avoid while you are taking guanfacine

Until you know for sure how guanfacine will affect you, it is best that you avoid getting behind the wheel of a car, operating heavy/hazardous machinery, or doing anything hazardous for a couple of weeks or so.

Guanfacine might cause your reflexes to slow down considerably, and impede your judgment making capabilities. This is why it is unsafe for you to drive a car or operate any heavy machinery.

You should also minimize, if not completely quit, drinking alcoholic beverages because it can increase the effects of guanfacine.

Side effects of guanfacine

You need to seek emergency medical help if you see any signs of allergic reaction, like breaking out in hives, labored breathing, and especially if any swelling occurs in your face, tongue, and lips.

- It is important to contact your doctor if you have:

- Severe anxiety and nervousness

- Sudden hallucinations

- Constant drowsiness

- Irregularly slow heart rate

- Feelings of extreme lightheadedness, like you are always on the verge of fainting

If for any reason you need to stop taking guanfacine, immediately call your doctor when you experience:

- Chronic headaches

- Confusion

- Increased heartbeat

- Involuntary shaking of your hands

- Raised blood pressure

If you leave these withdrawal symptoms untreated, they could lead to increased high blood pressure, blurry vision, or epileptic seizures.

Clonidine (Kapvay)

Clonidine can help lower blood pressure by decreasing the amounts of certain chemicals in your bloodstream. This allows the walls of the blood vessels to relax and let more blood flow through them, so the heart does not need to beat as hard anymore.

The Catapres brand of clonidine is used for treating hypertension, while the Kapvay brand is for treating ADHD.

Clonidine is sometimes taken in conjunction with other medications.

Important points

Before taking any form of clonidine, you need to inform your doctor if you are currently suffering from:

- Any kind of heart disease

- Heart arrhythmia

- Unusually slow heartbeat

- Low blood pressure

- If you have a history of stroke and/or heart attack

- Kidney disease

- Or if you have an allergic reaction to Catapres

Before you take clonidine

If you were found to be allergic to Catapres, then you should avoid taking any form of clonidine.

The jury is still out on whether clonidine has any negative effects on unborn babies, but you should still tell your doctor if you are pregnant, or if you are planning on getting pregnant in the near future.

Clonidine can pass through the mother's blood and into her breastmilk, and it might cause harm to a nursing baby. You need to talk with your doctor regarding clonidine if you are currently breastfeeding so that you can be prescribed with another, safer alternative.

How to take clonidine?

You should follow your doctor's instructions on the prescription note to the letter. You should never change the dosage amount; do not add or remove anything from your prescribed dosage.

Clonidine is usually taken in the morning and just before bedtime.

You can take clonidine with or without eating first.

You should not take two forms of clonidine at once. Aside from oral tablets and capsules, clonidine also comes in the form of transdermal patches.

When taking extended-release tablets, you need to swallow them whole. You should never crush, break apart, or chew on the tablet, as this will defeat it purpose of gradually releasing the clonidine into your bloodstream.

If you are needing surgery, regardless if it is a minor job, you need to tell your surgeon that you are currently using clonidine. You might need to stop using the medication a couple of days before and after the surgery.

It is dangerous to suddenly stop using clonidine as you will likely experience horrible withdrawal symptoms. If you really need to stop taking clonidine, consult with your doctor on how to safely do so with minimal withdrawal symptoms.

Contact your doctor when you are sick and are experiencing nausea and vomiting. Prolonged illness makes your body less reliable when it comes to absorbing clonidine, which may lead to withdrawal symptoms even if you are still following your dosage schedule.

What to do if you miss a dose?

You need to take the missed dose as soon as you remember, however, if your next scheduled dose is in less than an hour, just forget about your missed dose and take the next one on time. You should not take a double dosage of clonidine as it could lead to dependence, and overdosing.

What happens if you overdose?

If you accidentally take two doses of clonidine, do not panic. Seek emergency medical attention, or call the Poison Help line at 1-800-222-1222 for advice on what to do.

The symptoms of overdosing in clonidine, include, but are not limited to:

- Severe high blood pressure

- Nosebleeds

- Anxiety

- Chest pains

- Miosis, also known as excessive constriction of the pupils of the eyes

- Shortness of breath

What should you avoid while you are taking clonidine?

Minimize, if not completely eliminate, alcohol intake. Drinking alcoholic beverages tends to increase the severity and duration of certain side effects of clonidine.

Clonidine might impair your judgment and slow down your reflexes considerably. This is the reason why you should avoid driving or operating heavy machinery until you find out the extent of the effects that clonidine has on you.

Some people have reported experiencing severe drowsiness when they take clonidine, so it might be a good idea to avoid participating in risky activities for the time being.

Side effects of clonidine

If you notice signs of an allergic reaction due to your taking of clonidine, like breaking out in hives, difficulty breathing, and swelling in different parts of the face, then call emergency medical services.

You also need to inform your doctor if you notice the following symptoms:

- Chest pain

- Difficulty breathing

- Heart arrhythmia

- Severe headaches, which feels like there's someone pounding on your neck and behind the ear

- Frequent nosebleeds

- Lightheadedness

- Anxiety and severe confusion

- Always feeling as if you will faint any second

- Anxiety and confusion

The more serious side effects of clonidine are more likely to happen in older adults. Such side effects include:

- Constant drowsiness

- Chronic fatigue

- Irritability

- Cottonmouth and loss of appetite

- Constipation

- Sleeping problems like insomnia and night terrors

Therapy for ADHD

Other than taking medication, you can also use different kinds of therapy to treat ADHD in adults. The use of therapy is also found to be effective for treating other problems that are connected to ADHD, such as problems with conduct, or anxiety disorders.

Here are some of the forms of therapy that are currently being used for treating adult ADHD:

Psychoeducation

This is the process of educating people who are seeking, or are currently receiving, other types of mental health treatment.

What is the Purpose of Psychoeducation?

One of the end goals of psychoeducation is to help more people understand, and thus feel more comfortable with mental health conditions. This is also one of the most important parts of all therapy programs. In general, the people who thoroughly understand the challenges that they are currently living with, also know about their individual coping abilities, their internal and external resources, and their strengths, which make them more able to address these difficulties. A knowledge of the symptoms one is experiencing can help them to feel that they are in control, and that they have what it takes to work towards improving their mental and emotional well-being.

One study found that psychoeducation, when used on patients who were dealing with schizophrenia, helped to reduce their treatment fees, and the number of days that the person spent on average in the hospital. This is why psychoeducation is also a vital part of most trauma therapies.

Most of the people who have a mental condition, like ADHD, know little or nothing at all about their ailment. The problem here is that they might have incorrect expectations about the therapy, or of the positive and negative effects of their medications. Even if they were given ample reading material by their doctors, the technical terms in them often only serve to confuse them even more instead of actually being helpful.

Psychoeducation can be either through one-on-one sessions, or with a group. This form of therapy not only benefits the patient, but also his/her parents and family, friends, and caregivers. This is not exactly a "treatment" per se, but it is one of the important first steps of getting treatment, because it offers all of the individuals involved in caring for the patient information on how to support them, and also how to maintain their own emotional health and their own well-being. This also provides them the chance to fully understand the mental health issues of their loved ones.

The Process of Psychoeducation

Psychoeducation might be general, or it can be highly specific, and it can be dispensed in a number of different ways. However, it is steered by four main goals: transference of information, support for medication and treatment, for training and support in self-help and self-care, and the creation of a safe space where one can vent any emotional frustration.

The following are components of psychoeducation:

- The therapist explaining to the patient the many ways that mental illness can affect normal functions.

- A psychiatrist explaining how prescribed medication can help patients deal with the symptoms of a mental illness.

- A psychiatric clinic providing support and education to the family of people who have mental illnesses like ADHD.

- Formal classes that are meant to educate the public about specific mental illnesses and mental health in general.

- Professional behavioral management support for students with ADHD and other mental illnesses that affect their behavior.

- Support groups that are meant to encourage people with mental illnesses to share experiences, strategies, and important information about their illness with each other.

- Some people receive psychoeducation through other means, like DVDs, audio CDs, online videos, and other audiovisual materials. However, there are still some that prefer to participate in sessions with a professional.

How Can Psychoeducation Help You?

Regardless of whether psychoeducation is dispensed in a clinic, school, or hospital, or through the phone or online, it more often than not leads to increased compliance of people to treatment regimens. When people who have been diagnosed with ADHD understand what their diagnosis means, it is more likely that they will view their condition as a treatable illness rather than something to be ashamed of.

When the family is involved in psychoeducation, it can also increase compliance as it also ensures that the patient receives enough emotional support while they receive treatment.

In addition to helping the patients diagnosed with ADHD understand their condition better, psychoeducation also helps in defeating the stigma surrounding mental health issues. There are now organizations like the National Alliance on Mental Illness (NAMI) that are advocating for increasing the amount of psychoeducation that consumers of mental health services and their families receive.

The more people know about mental health issues, specifically the fact that mental illnesses are not the results of bad choices, the more likely they will be to be accepting of people with mental illnesses.

Behavior therapy

This is an umbrella term that encompasses all types of therapy that are used for treating mental illnesses. This type of therapy aims to identify potentially self-destructive behaviors and then help to change them. Behavior therapy functions on the idea that all behaviors are acquired, and that unhealthy behaviors can be reformed. The main goal of this treatment is to diagnose current problems and create plans for changing them.

Who Benefits from Behavioral Therapy?

This type of therapy can help people who are suffering from a wide array of mental disorders. People most commonly seek behavioral therapy to find solutions for:

- Anger management

- Excessive panic disorders

- Anxiety disorders

- Depression

Behavioral therapy can also be used for treating:

- Post-traumatic stress disorder (PTSD)

- Bipolar disorder

- Different kinds of phobias

- Obsessive-compulsive disorder

- Self-harming

* Substance abuse

* And of course, Attention Deficit Hyperactivity Disorder (ADHD)

Different Types of Behavioral Therapy

There are different kinds of behavioral therapy, and they focus on different parts of a person's psyche.

Cognitive Behavioral Therapy (CBT)

CBT is quite possibly the most popular form of behavioral therapy. CBT combines traditional behavioral therapy with cognitive therapy. The treatment focuses on how the person's thoughts and beliefs can influence their actions and moods. CBT commonly focuses on current problems and looks for solutions for them. However, the long-term goal of Cognitive Behavioral Therapy is to alter a person's unhealthy way of thinking and behavior into a productive and healthier one.

This form of therapy is commonly used to help people with ADHD cope with their symptoms, and somewhat lessen their effects.

Cognitive Behavioral Play Therapy

As the name implies, this form of behavioral therapy is commonly used on child patients. The therapists can gain useful insights into the things that children have trouble saying, or cannot express, just by watching them play. The kids are allowed to choose their own toys and play as they would normally. The therapists might ask the kids to draw a picture, or using toys, recreate a scene. The therapists can also teach the parents techniques on how they can use their children's playtimes to improve their communication.

System Desensitization

This is a form of therapy that is usually used to treat phobias. System desensitization builds its foundation on classical mental conditioning. The therapists teach people to replace a fear response with relaxation responses; like breathing techniques. Once the patient masters this, the therapist will expose them to gradually increasing amounts of the things that the patient fears. The gradual introduction of the phobias allows the patient to practice relaxation techniques without getting overwhelmed with fear.

Aversion Therapy

This type of behavioral therapy is commonly used for treating problems like alcoholism and drug addiction. The way this therapy works is somewhat the opposite of System Desensitization; the therapist teaches the patient to associate a stimulus that he usually finds desirable, but is unhealthy, with an unpleasant stimulus, preferably something that causes discomfort for the patient. For instance, the therapist can teach the patient to associate the smell of alcohol with an unpleasant memory.

Is Behavioral Therapy Effective?

Yes, behavioral therapy is actually extremely effective in treating mental disorders. Hundreds of thousands of people, maybe even millions, have successfully used behavioral therapy to turn their lives around and actually become productive individuals.

Ideally, a treatment program for ADHD will take a multi-faceted approach that combines multiple methods of treatment, including behavioral therapy.

Chapter 4 – Alternative ADHD Treatments

Although the proven way to treat adult ADHD is through a combination of medication and therapy, some people are not too thrilled about using drugs as a coping mechanism. For them, not only is the risk of addiction all too real, the side effects that come with most ADHD medications are nothing to sneeze at. This is why there are a lot of people who are looking into alternative forms of treatment in the hopes that they can find solace without taking any huge risks.

A word of warning though, not just because something is "100% natural" that does not mean that it is completely safe; you still have to check if you are allergic to anything you take.

Dietary Supplements

Although just adding more vitamins and minerals into your diet will not cure you of ADHD, they definitely can help make dealing with the symptoms much easier. With today's busy lifestyle, it is safe to assume that you might not be eating the right kinds of foods all the time. Also, considering your condition, finding the time and the energy to cook your own food can be difficult, which is why you may often eat out or have food delivered to you.

According to research conducted by a researcher from the Child and Adolescent Psychiatric Clinics of North America, the following mineral supplements show promise in helping with the treatment of ADHD in both children and adults:

Melatonin

This substance is usually used for helping treat insomnia and other sleep disorders. Melatonin does not seem to have any direct impact on ADHD symptoms itself. However, sleeping disorders can make the symptoms of ADHD worse, so improving your sleep by using melatonin can be an effective strategy.

Scientists have gathered enough significant evidence to show that there is a very close association between ADHD and sleep disorders. They suggest that possibly, disruptions in normal circadian rhythms may have something to do with the two conditions.

With that said, taking supplements will help balance your melatonin levels, and because melatonin is responsible for your wake-sleep cycle, this will help you deal with insomnia, and in effect ADHD as well.

Vitamin C

The brain uses Vitamin C — drawn out of the blood and cycled through the brain — to make neurotransmitters like dopamine and norepinephrine. Foods such as oranges, red peppers, and kale are high in Vitamin C, but it's also possible to take a daily supplement if nutritional changes aren't enough. However, Vitamin C can interfere with the absorption of ADHD medication, so it should not be taken an hour before or after administering ADHD medication.

Iron

Past research has linked iron deficiency in infancy to slower brain development and poorer school performance later in childhood. Animal studies have also linked iron deficiency to abnormal muscle movement or restlessness. Iron deficiency is also common in people with the movement disorder known as restless legs syndrome.

The children with the most severe iron deficiencies were also the most inattentive, impulsive, and hyperactive. This led the researchers to conclude that "low iron stores may explain as much as 30% of ADHD severity."

The researchers say the reason for the low iron levels in children with ADHD is unclear. The children in the study did not have evidence of malnutrition, which might contribute to low iron levels.

Zinc

Some studies suggest that children with ADHD may have lower levels of zinc in their bodies. In addition, some scientists have reported that children with the disorder who took zinc supplements along with traditional ADHD treatment showed improvement in their symptoms.

Several studies have shown a drop in hyperactivity and impulsivity with zinc supplements. The same research, though, reports no change in inattentiveness, which is another key symptom of ADHD. A 2005 study in the Journal of Child and Adolescent Psychopharmacology, though, did show a link between zinc levels and teacher- and parent-rated inattention in children.

Magnesium

Magnesium supplements with vitamin B6, which increases magnesium absorption, have shown promise for reducing ADHD symptoms. One study found that 58% of participants with ADHD had low serum magnesium levels. All of the children were given preparations of magnesium plus vitamin B6, 100 mg/day, for a period of 1 to 6 months. In all of the children, physical aggression, instability, attention at school, muscle rigidity, spasms, and twitching improved.

One of the children treated was a six-year-old referred to as "J." Initially he suffered from aggressiveness, anxiety, inattention, and a lack of self-control. After taking the magnesium plus vitamin B6 supplements for 6 months, he experienced better sleep and concentration—and no methylphenidate was needed (Mousain-Bosc et al., 2004).

Vitamin B

Deficiencies in B vitamins — particularly B6 — can cause irritability and fatigue in children and adults with ADHD. Adequate B6 levels — achieved through nutritional changes or a supplement — can increase alertness and decrease anxiety-like symptoms. Foods high in B6 include wild-caught tuna, bananas, spinach, and salmon.

Omega-3

Now evidence is showing that omega-3 fatty acids help to optimize brain function. Among other things, omega-3s boost the body's synthesis of dopamine, the neurotransmitter that ADHD medications act to increase.

So, could a daily fish oil capsule help curb the symptoms of ADHD?

Quite possibly, suggest several research studies on fish oil for ADHD — including a study published in Pediatrics. "A lack of certain polyunsaturated fatty acids may contribute to dyslexia and attention-deficit/hyperactivity disorder," reports one of the study's authors, Paul Montgomery, D.Phil., a researcher in the psychiatry department at the University of Oxford in England.

Carnitine

Often used in the treatment of ADHD, carnitine can help boost the effectiveness of omega-3s, improve memory, and play a role in the synthesis of dopamine. It also can improve behavioral problems like aggression and hyperactivity. Also, many individuals with ADHD have glucose deficiencies that inhibit the uptake of carnitine into the brain. Hence, supplementing with carnitine is believed to help increase the energy production in the mitochondria.

The use of any medication, including supplements, carries some risk. Children, in particular, should not take any supplementary or complementary medicine without their doctor's approval.

Most supplements do not have approval from the U.S. Food and Drug Administration (FDA). As a result, there is no regulation on the contents, and no official recommended dosage.

People must always check with a doctor whether it is safe to use a supplement or other remedy, and what dosage they should take.

Herbal medicines

Clinical trials have found that a number of herbal treatments may show promise for treating ADHD. These include:

Gotu Kola

This herbal remedy has been in use for centuries by many Asian cultures as a treatment for skin diseases, and also to improve brain function. It is widely believed to stimulate the mind by lessening anxiety, and at the same time increasing mental alertness.

Clinical tests found that gotu kola is also a mild antibacterial, adaptogen, anti-inflammatory, and anti-viral to a certain degree. It is also an anxiolytic, stimulates the circulatory system, and is a cerebral tonic.

Ginseng

Ginseng, is an herbal remedy that has been used for centuries in China. This medicinal plant has a myriad of medicinal properties, which is why it is quite expensive, and also why it is so popular. One of the supposed illnesses that ginseng, particularly the red ginseng variety, can help with is ADHD.

In 2011, a study was conducted on 18 children, aged 6 to 14 years old, and all of whom were diagnosed with ADHD. The test subjects were given 1000mg of ginseng daily for eight weeks. After the trial period, the children had reportedly significant improvements in terms of their anxiety, behavior, and social functioning.

French Maritime Pine (Pycnogenol)

Pycnogenol is an extract taken from the bark of the French maritime pine. This herbal remedy is said to have potent effects when it comes to treating ADHD, and this claim is backed by several independent studies.

In one study, the researchers gave 61 children either 1mg of pycnogenol, or a similar amount of placebo (this is the control group) once a day for four weeks. Only the researchers knew who got what. After the trial period, the researchers found that the pycnogenol group had significantly less hyperactivity as compared to the control group which showed no improvement whatsoever.

In another study, the researchers found out that the pycnogenol extract helped balance the antioxidant levels of the children diagnosed with ADHD. In yet another study, which was published in 2007, pycnogenol extract was found to help lower the amounts of stress hormones by more than 25%, and decreased the amount of dopamine by more than 10% in people who were diagnosed with ADHD.

Lemon Balm

Lemon balm is usually consumed as a relaxing tea, but it also has other medicinal properties, some of which are beneficial to treating ADHD. Lemon balm is more popularly known for its antiviral and antibacterial properties, but it also has anxiolytic properties, which means it can soothe the nerves and helps reduce stress. The compound in lemon balm that is responsible for its calming effect is rosmarinic acid, a substance that inhibits the release of GABA transaminase, an enzyme that metabolizes gamma-Aminobutyric acid (GABA). Low GABA levels are linked to ADHD.

People diagnosed with ADHD who consume lemon balm reported that they experienced better moods and much improved mental performance. Eugenol, yet another active ingredient in lemon balm, is also a muscle relaxant, and has a mild analgesic property that produces a numbing and relaxing sensation throughout the body; this greatly helps minimize hyperactivity.

Red Clover

Also known as sweet clover, red clover is said to help relieve the symptoms of ADHD because it has the ability to reduce depression and eliminate certain mood disorders in people diagnosed with ADHD. The substance in red clover that is responsible for all these benefits is the chemical transcischloramide, which is a precursor to dopamine production.

Dopamine is a neurotransmitter that plays a vital role in many brain functions, and unfortunately also plays a huge role in the symptoms displayed by ADHD. When there is too much dopamine in an ADHD patient's system, it causes them to become fidgety, impulsive, and find it difficult to focus on a single task for more than a couple of minutes before getting distracted. Aside from treating ADHD symptoms, red clover can also be helpful in treating respiratory infections, wounds, and it also holds some promise in regulating blood sugar levels in people suffering from diabetes.

Rhodiola

Rhodiola rosea is an adaptogenic herb that has shown quite some promise in improving the ability to focus in both children and adults diagnosed with ADHD. Rhodiola has also been used in many Asian cultures as a means to fight against fatigue and improve a person's memory.

The way rhodiola works is that it increases the sensitivity of the body's neurological and nervous systems, which are the ones that are responsible for the production of serotonin and dopamine. The reduction of these two brain chemicals can greatly improve the symptoms of ADHD.

Passion Flower

This herb is highly recommended by traditional herbalists as a potent treatment for ADHD symptoms. Passion flower has the capabilities to even out a person's mood swings, and in the process improve their concentration. In addition, according to a study published in the Journal of Clinical pharmacy and Therapeutics, passion flower has several benefits that can help to improve generalized anxiety disorder.

Eleuthero

Also called Siberian ginseng, eleuthero is among the most popularly known herbal remedies that are used for ADHD. This helps in dealing with the symptoms associated with inattentive ADHD because it helps increase the person's awareness, and also can improve memory.

In one of the recent meetings of the American Stroke Association, a team of in-house researchers presented their findings of a recent study that they conducted. The research involved two groups of people, one group were given supplements containing eleuthero, and the other, which served as the control, were given placebos. The researchers found that the group that received the eleuthero actually showed a drastic improvement in their memory, while the participants who received placebos showed no significant improvement whatsoever.

Traditional herbalists have long known about the immune system boosting properties of eleuthero, and also its ability to help the body deal with stress.

Green Oats

Green oats are just regular oats that have not had enough time to ripen before they were harvested. They are commonly sold under the name "avena sativa". Herbalists have long known about the nerve-calming, and anxiety and stress-reducing properties of sativa.

Early studies have discovered that sativa extract has the ability to boost an ADHD sufferer's attention and concentration. In addition, a 2011 study discovered that when people took sativa extract, they made fewer mistakes on tests measuring their ability to focus on a task. A separate study also found that cognitive performance greatly improved when people took avena sativa supplements.

Bacopa Monnieri

Bacopa monnieri has for years only been traditionally prescribed by Ayurvedic healers to improve cognitive functions like focus, concentration, mental fortitude, and memory. Now, modern science has found that there might be some truth to the rumors about Bacopa. Research has found that Bacopa is a strong anxiolytic, meaning it can help fight the symptoms of anxiety and help boost a person's mood.

CBD Oil

Cannabidiol oil (CBD oil) is fast becoming one of the most popular treatment methods for different disorders like depression, anxiety, and ADHD; researchers have actually documented CBD as a worthwhile alternative to certain pharmaceutical medications.

The way CBD oil works is that it helps the endocannabinoid system of the body to work more efficiently. The endocannabinoid system modulates the functions of the brain, and the endocrine and immune systems. It mainly regulates the production of certain hormones that are related to reproduction, and how the body responds to stressors.

As the name implies, CBD oil comes from the cannabis plant, just like the psychoactive drug THC. However, unlike THC, CBD is not psychoactive in the least. It will not alter your mind at all when you use it. It has all the benefits, and more, without the psychoactive properties of THC.

Precautions about herbal medications

Just because something is "100% natural" does not mean it is completely safe to use. Keep in mind that hemlock, nightshade, and toadstools are all natural as well, but it is not safe to ingest them. You should treat herbal remedies just as you would pharmaceutical medications; you need to be careful when taking them.

There are still a lot of unknown variables when it comes to medicinal herbs. For instance, researchers are still looking into the actual effective dosage amounts of most herbal remedies. Studies are also still underway on whether or not medicinal herbs have negative interactions with other, known pharmaceutical medications.

Just to be on the safe side, if you get a recommendation for a medicinal herb supplement from someone you know, consult first with your doctor. You never know if that herbal remedy might have negative interactions with the medications that you are already using. In addition, the herbal supplements might contain substances that you may be allergic to.

Chapter 5 – Managing Adult ADHD

Although there is no known cure for ADHD at the moment, that does not mean that you have to suffer for the rest of your life. Aside from medication, therapy, and healthy lifestyle changes, there are also strategies for managing your ADHD symptoms so you can live a healthy and normal life.

The Stigma Attached to Adult ADHD

There is no shame in having Attention Deficit Hyperactivity Disorder. However, because society is the way it is, people who have ADHD are often seen as someone who's "defective", and this is despite ample evidence that suggests that they can just be as competent and skilled as everyone else.

Why is there stigma attached to having ADHD?

Even though there are mountains of empirical evidence that proves its existence, there are still many people who do not believe that ADHD is a bona fide health issue. They see people with ADHD as simply lazy or sloppy; and the fact that the symptoms of ADHD seem to randomly come and go, somehow reinforces their incorrect perceptions.

Another factor that contributes to the stigma surrounding ADHD is the opinions of people regarding the use of psychiatric drugs. In recent years, there is a surge in the number of people who are taking medication to deal with their ADHD, and some people are wondering if those people actually do have a reason to take said drugs, or if they just say they do so they can have access to them.

Finally, society seems to think that when you have poor academic performance that you are not worth your salt. This is especially damaging when people are not even aware of the reason why the person's grades are so low, which is quite often the case with ADHD.

What Harm Does the Stigmatization of ADHD Cause?

The most obvious things that the stigmatization of ADHD, or any kind of mental illness in general, can bring are social problems and discrimination in the workplace. Some of the social problems that come with the stigmatization of ADHD include being told that you do not have a real issue; you are just lazy and unmotivated. What people do not know is that no matter how hard someone with ADHD "applies himself", he can only do so for short bursts, and it can be mentally exhausting for the person.

However, the biggest harm caused by the stigmatization of ADHD might not actually come from other people, but from the sufferer himself. It is when people with ADHD internalize the negative stereotypes about them that they do the most damage.

It is quite saddening to see children with ADHD say things like, "I'm not cut out for school anyway," or "I'm no good at this kind of thing". The stigma surrounding ADHD has corrupted their young minds so much that they no longer have any motivation to achieve anything; they have already given up on trying to be successful academically.

The flipside of self-stigmatization, which is denial, may be just as destructive as its counterpart. This is when you consider the stereotypes surrounding ADHD and you refuse to believe that you fall into them. You do not want to be associated with a condition that you consider as very shameful, and you firmly believe that that is not who you really are.

People who have ADHD find it difficult to look at themselves realistically, and their strong desire to distance themselves from the illness makes it almost impossible to accept that they have it. Here's an example: you refuse to take medication even though your physician told you that it would help you control the symptoms of ADHD, because you believe in your heart of hearts that if you take medication you are admitting that you have a problem. You actually believe that by not taking medication you are invalidating the diagnosis of ADHD. Sadly, this is a common occurrence.

The stigma of ADHD is a difficult burden for everyone, but it seems that girls and young women are carrying a heavier load. Society tends to think that ADHD is a disorder that affects only boys, so when a girl is diagnosed with ADHD it can be a hard thing for people to fathom.

Adults also have to deal with the same kind of stereotyping, as most people think that ADHD is a kids-only thing; like it's a phase that people eventually grow out of. When an adult then admits to having ADHD, he or she is immediately put under scrutiny, or are stereotyped.

How to Deal with ADHD's Stigma

What should you do when someone says something hurtful about your ADHD? It is all too easy to just feel hurt and turn away, or maybe give the other person a good tongue-lashing, but the best course of action is to have a gentle, yet firm, discussion with the person. Inform him or her that their opinion of your condition is archaic and that you take offense over what the person has said. Continue by informing the person of the things that you have to endure on a daily basis, that the simple things that he or she takes for granted are actually quite challenging for you.

Raising awareness instead of arguing with people who have the wrong idea about ADHD is the better course of action.

What else can you do to counter the effects of ADHD stereotyping? When you are more aware of the stereotypes surrounding your condition, it will be easier to recognize when they are affecting you.

In addition, you also need to recognize when the negative feedback you are getting is actually valid. Do not think that all the feedback you are getting is the result of negative stereotyping. You do still have to take responsibility for your behavior and actions, and not simply use your diagnosis as an excuse.

Another way to prevent the stereotyping of ADHD from affecting you is by taking positive action. Joining other people who share the same plight as you to end discrimination is very empowering.

You should also consider joining ADHD advocacy groups if you have not already done so. There are many groups that you can join, like CHADD and ADDA. You can also get in touch with your local elected representative and ask if he or she could take action that could benefit the ADHD community.

How and When Should You Reveal That You Have ADHD?

This can be quite a conundrum. The reason why you are concealing the fact that you have been diagnosed with ADHD is because you want to avoid being labeled as such, and also so you can avoid the discrimination that often comes with the condition.

So, when should you tell your boss, your new friends, and the other people who do not know about your diagnosis? With regards to your boss, it will depend on their disposition. If your employer has a reputation of being very open and accommodating, then there should not be any problem telling them whenever you can. However, if you're not sure about how your boss will react, the best policy is always to be up-front. Don't hesitate to let them know, particularly if you think your ADHD will affect how you act and perform in the workplace.

It may not be necessary that everyone in your life knows about your ADHD. However, if you think that your ADHD is affecting your relationship with a friend or loved one, it's always best to let them know so that they can be more understanding. Remember, secrecy will only fan the feelings of shame. It is better if you seek out people whom you feel comfortable telling your secret to, open up, and be receptive to their advice.

Tips for Getting Organized and Controlling Clutter

The trademarks of people with ADHD are an inability to focus, and being easy to distract, which makes organization one of the biggest challenges that adults with ADHD have to face. If you have been recently diagnosed with ADHD, just looking at all the clutter and mess in your home might make you feel overwhelmed, mainly because you do not know how or where to begin.

Learning to break your larger tasks into smaller "sub-tasks" and develop and follow a simple system to organize will make things easier. Making use of different routines and structures is essential in keeping organized. Also, make use of all available tools at your disposal such as daily planners and setting reminders. By implementing these strategies to help you stay organized, you will be well on your way to having an organized and clutter-free home.

Develop Structure and Neatness Habits; and Keep on Doing Them

To start organizing a room, begin by separating the clutter into different categories. Basically, you will be deciding which of the things you still need, which of them you can stow away, and which of them you can throw out. To organize yourself, get into the habit of making lists and keeping a small notebook with you so you can take notes whenever you need to. You need to maintain your new habits and structures by turning them into your regular routines; basically, making them part of your daily life until you begin doing them automatically without even thinking.

Create/Set aside space for storage – You need to ask yourself what are the things that you need daily, and then create space for these things to exist in your home. For instance, place a bowl on your nightstand or on the side table beside the front door for things like your keys, wallet, loose change, and all of the things that you need, but usually misplace. Also, place a small waste basket nearby so you can throw away the things in your pockets that you do not need anymore, like ticket stubs, receipts, wrappers, and other miscellaneous stuff that you might have.

Make use of a calendar app or a daily planner – Whether you like using cutting edge technology, or if you want to keep it old school, there are tools that you can use to keep organized. You can use the calendar app on your smartphone or computer to help you remember important dates and appointments; you can even set up alarms that will remind you days in advance to make sure that you do not forget. You can also get yourself a smart watch that you can sync with your smartphone, so you do not even have to open your smartphone, the reminders will be sent straight to your wrist.

Learn to create and use lists and notes – You can use lists and notes to better keep track of your regular tasks, ongoing projects, upcoming deadlines, and if you have any appointments that day. If you choose to use an old school day planner, keep your lists inside it so you will not lose them. If you go with the smartphone route, you can make use of "to-do" apps.

Deal with the clutter right now – One of the best ways to deal with clutter and avoid forgetfulness and procrastination is to deal with it right away. File papers as soon as you see them, clean up small messes immediately, and return phone calls and messages as soon as you are reminded of them. If a task does not take more than two minutes to do, then do it right away instead of later. This is a habit that you can develop, and over time you will find yourself procrastinating less.

Regain control of your paper trail

Dealing with paperwork can be quite a big hurdle when you are suffering from ADHD, and this might be a huge part of your disorganization. But what if I told you that you can put an end to the seemingly endless piles of paper cluttering your kitchen counter, nightstand, or office desk? All that you need to do is set aside some time to create a paperwork sorting system that works for you.

Sort your mail daily – All you will need are a few minutes to sort through the various mail that you get on a daily basis, and you can start right after you take it out of the mailbox, or at a specific time every day. It will help immensely if you have a place that is dedicated just for mail, preferably one that has different compartments; one for filing, one for immediate action, and one for those that should go straight to the trash.

Go paperless – These days, it is possible to just ask your billers to send you an electronic copy of your bills via email. This way, you are essentially killing two birds with one stone; you are getting rid of most of the paper clutter that you have to go through, and you are also doing your part to help the environment.

Start a filing system – Make use of file dividers, or use separate folders for different important documents, like medical records, receipts, income statements, and coupons. Clearly label and color-code each folder so the next time that you need to find something, you will find it much faster.

Tips for time management and how to never miss a deadline again

People with ADHD struggle constantly with time management. It is quite easy for them to lose track of time, procrastinate, and underestimate the amount of time that they actually need to complete their tasks. Or maybe they are doing things in an illogical order.

Many adults with ADHD often fall into the trap of spending so much time on a single task that nothing else gets done, and this is known as "hyper-focusing". These kinds of problems often make you feel very frustrated with yourself, and you might even feel impatient. However, there are ways that you can teach yourself to make the most use of your time and improve your work efficiency exponentially.

Time management tips

For an adult with ADHD, the passage of time can seem very different from other people. For instance, if you are tasked with a huge, redundant task, the passage of time may seem to be very slow. On the other hand, when you are doing something that interests you, time seems to fly by so fast. To calibrate yourself with other people, you can simply use the oldest trick in the book, wear a watch.

Turn into a clock-watcher – Wear a wristwatch all the time or, have a very visible wall clock or desk clock so you can see how much time has passed since you started on a task. When starting on a task, take note of the time. You may want to even physically write down the time so that you don't forget when you started.

Use countdown timers – Only give yourself a limited amount of time for each task, and then set an alarm to play a tune or sound whenever the time is up. If you are working on a larger task, set up several alarms that will go off at regular intervals so you are constantly alerted and reminded to work on your task.

Give yourself more time for tasks – If you are like most other adults with ADHD, you are very bad at estimating timelines; you find it hard to even come up with a ballpark figure of how much time you will need to do something. You will need to create a bumper number so that you will actually have more than enough time for things. For instance, if you think it will only take you thirty minutes to go grocery shopping, add another ten to twenty minutes to your estimate and you will be good to go.

Plan to be early, and constantly remind yourself of your plan – When setting appointments, act as if they are at least fifteen minutes earlier than the actual time that you need to meet. Set up additional alarms to remind you to get ready and leave the house on time. This will make sure that you will not be frantically running around the house and wasting a lot of precious time because you cannot find your keys or your phone.

Tips for prioritizing

Adults with ADHD often struggle at controlling their impulses and tend to jump from one task to another. Most often, both tasks are totally unrelated, and in the end neither task actually gets completed. This makes it difficult for people with ADHD to complete, or even just attempt to finish large tasks. Here are a few strategies to help combat this bad habit:

Decide on what to do first – Ask yourself, which task on your list is the most important, which is the second most important, and so on.

Take one step at a time – For larger jobs, break them into smaller, more manageable steps. For a simple example, if the large task is to "peel and slice a pineapple", you can break it down further into individual steps, like "cut off the top with the leaves", then "chop off the bottom", and then "allow the pineapple to stand, and using a large kitchen knife, take off the hard outer skin of the pineapple", and so on. This might seem like a silly example, but the same process can be applied to practically and task you need to complete, particularly if it first appears to be large and daunting.

Keep your eyes on the task – Avoid getting distracted by only working on the tasks in your schedule, and maybe even use a timer so you can concentrate better on finishing said task. Remove all distractions from the room, and perhaps even create a dedicated workspace where you will do any important tasks.

Learn when it is okay to say no

If you are more affected by the impulsive symptoms of ADHD, then you might have a problem with agreeing to work on too many projects or saying yes to too many social events. It does not matter if you can manage to cram everything into your schedule, because that in itself is the problem; just looking at a packed schedule can make you feel really overwhelmed. And by not giving yourself enough time to work on tasks, you sacrifice the quality of your work. The next time someone asks you to do something for them, check your schedule first, and say no if there simply is no room in it. Using a calendar app on your smartphone is a great way to keep a track of your schedule. Set one up and make it a habit to check the schedule before agreeing to anything, no matter how small!

Tips for managing money and bills

Proper money management requires skills in budgeting, organization, planning, and lots of self-discipline, which means that it can be quite a challenge for adults with ADHD. Unfortunately, conventional money management techniques do not usually work for adults with ADHD, mainly because they require a lot of time and attention to detail, of which they are in short supply. However, if you create your own money managing system that is both simple and consistent, you will be able to get a good grip on your finances and stop your overspending habits.

Controlling your budget

Making an honest assessment of your current financial situation is the first step in controlling your budget. You can start by keeping a close eye on your every expense, regardless of how small it is, for a month. This will give you a good idea on where your money is going monthly. After monitoring your expenses, you might be surprised at just how much money you are wasting on impulse purchases.

Using your expenditures as a guide, you can then create a monthly budget that can cover all your needs and some of your wants. There are plenty of budgeting apps and computer programs that can help to simplify this process.

Figure out a system to prevent you from straying away from the budget that you set out for yourself. For instance, if you find that you have been spending way too much money eating at restaurants, you can prepare an eating-in plan and factor in some time for going grocery shopping and cooking your own meals. Planning things out in advance is vital in budgeting successfully if you have ADHD.

Setting up an idiot-proof money management and bill paying system

You need to make an easy, yet organized system that will help you file your receipts and stay on top of your bills. For an adult with ADHD, online banking is heaven sent. Organizing your finances online means you no longer have to deal with stacks of paperwork, misplaced invoices, messy handwriting, or any other issue that arises when dealing with paperwork.

Balancing your budget on your own can be a hit-or-miss affair, but it will all change once you switch over to online banking. Your online bank account will give you access to all of the deposits and withdrawals that you made, which makes tracking your balance a lot more convenient. You can keep track of every penny that you spend every day.

In addition, through online banking, you can set up the automatic payment of your monthly bills, as well as log in and pay through your account as needed for any irregular expenses that might have come up unexpectedly. This means that you no longer have to stress about misplaced envelopes and no more paying of late fees.

On the other hand, if you prefer not to pay your bills automatically, bill payments can still be made easier using electronic reminders. You can either set them up as a text or email reminder through your online banking account, or you can set them into your schedule using your smartphone's calendar app.

There are many free online services that can help you keep track of your finances and bank accounts. They will take a bit of time and effort to set up properly, but once you have linked your bank accounts, they will automatically update. These tools can really make your (financial) life much easier.

Tips for staying focused and productive at work

The professional world is stressful enough as it is, and having ADHD just adds a whole set of extra challenges. To make things worse, the things that you are tasked to do the entire day, like completing tasks, organizing files, sitting still and listening quietly, are all the things that you likely have the most trouble with.

Having ADHD and making sure that you still do a stellar job is not an easy task, but if you do a bit of tweaking to your workplace you can take advantage of your strengths and at the same time minimize the effects of your ADHD symptoms.

Getting Organized at Work

Just like what you did at home, you need to take it slow when organizing your desk, cubicle, or office at work. You can implement the following strategies to make sure that your workplace stays clean and with everything in its rightful place:

Set aside some time daily for organization – Having a messy desk can be distracting, which is the bane of people who have ADHD. You do not need to organize things all in one go; you just need to set aside maybe five or ten minutes of your time before you start working, or you can do it right before you clock out. You will still get paid for your time, and just by setting some time aside for organizing, your efficiency will drastically improve.

Use lists and color-code them if possible – By writing a to-do list before you start working, you will lessen the chances of you forgetting anything. Color-coding your lists will also prove handy as this system will make it easier for you to focus on the things that you need to prioritize; and speaking of prioritizing...

Prioritize your tasks – When making your to-do list, you need to put the tasks that are the most important right at the top. This way you will remember to do them before starting on any of the low-priority tasks. You should also impose a deadline on everything that you do. Doing so will make you actually want to start on your list.

Getting Rid of Distractions

Keeping focus on your work is hard enough when you have ADHD, if there are things that distract you while you are at work then getting things done might seem impossible. Aside from letting your co-workers know that you would appreciate it if they do not disturb you while you are working, here are some techniques that you can use to minimize workplace distractions:

Where you work matters – If you do not have your own office, ask your boss if you could work in the conference room when no one is using it. During meetings, sit close to the speaker and avoid sitting next to the people who you know are chatty during meetings.

Minimize outside distractions – If possible, turn your desk so that it is facing against a wall so you will not get distracted by all the people walking about.

In addition, you should make it a point to not check your emails, social media, and voice mail until your break; and if it is not essential to your work, you should log off the internet altogether. If you are easily distracted by noise, use noise-cancelling headphones and play white noise out of them, or some lo-fi music to help you concentrate better.

Save your diabolical plans for later – If there's one good thing about having a hyperactive brain, it's that of the thousands of thoughts that seem to run through it, there are bound to be a couple that are actually viable.

However, instead of acting on them immediately, and distracting yourself from your tasks, jot your great ideas down on a small notebook or a piece of paper and then check on it later after work. Some people with ADHD enjoy scheduling some time after office hours that is devoted solely to going through their notes.

Increasing Your Attention Span

Adults with ADHD can focus on their tasks, it's just that they have a hard time maintaining that focus, especially when their tasks are repetitive and not at all interesting. For instance, boring meetings and office lectures can be hard on anyone, but they are particularly torturous for adults with ADHD. Also, keeping track of multiple instructions can be a bit difficult for people with ADHD.

If you want to improve your ability to focus, the following tips might help:

Get a written copy if possible – If you will be attending a meeting, seminar, a "talk", or any other kind of professional gathering, ask the organizer if you can have an advance copy of relevant materials, like a meeting agenda, outline, or anything similar. You can use these materials as a guide for active listening and note taking. Jotting down notes while you listen to the person speaking will help you focus more on the speaker's words.

Repeat any instructions you get – When the speaker gives verbal instructions, repeat them out loud, but in a more questioning manner, as if you are clarifying the instructions. Repeating instructions and directions will help you remember them more vividly later.

Get up and move about – No, this does not mean you can just stand up and leave in the middle of the lecture or meeting. Of course, you need to find the appropriate time and place for doing so. If you will not be disturbing anyone, you can squeeze a stress ball under your desk, or use a fidget spinner to keep your hands busy. If there is a bit of a break in the middle of talks, then take this opportunity to get out of the auditorium or meeting room, so you can stretch your legs and even jump up and down a bit. Get it all out of your system so you feel free and lighter later when the meeting resumes.

Tips For Managing Stress And Boosting Mood

Because of the impulsivity and disorganization that often comes with ADHD, you might also be burdened with other problems that are brought about by the symptoms of this condition, like problems with sleeping, eating unhealthily, or not getting enough physical exercise. These, in turn, can lead to crippling stress, crazy mood swings, and feeling overwhelmed by your own thoughts.

The best way that you can break free from this unhealthy cycle is to take charge and replace your unhealthy habits with new, much healthier, routines.

Living a healthier lifestyle, like eating healthy foods, getting ample amounts of sleep, and exercising regularly can help you stay calm and focused on your tasks. Healthier habits can help significantly reduce the impact and severity of ADHD symptoms like the inability to focus your attention for long periods, lack of energy, and others.

Exercise and Spending Time Outdoors

Getting enough exercise may be the most efficient way to manage the hyperactivity and inattentiveness brought about by ADHD. Some of the benefits brought about by exercise include:

- Relieves stress

- Boosts your mood

- Calms the mind

- Helps you use up all your excess energy

- Helps you release your aggression, which leads to more harmonious personal relationships, and also gives you a feeling of stability

Exercise every day – It does not matter what kind of exercise you do, as long as it is vigorous and fun so that you do not have to force yourself to do it. For instance, you could play basketball with your work friends every day at the end of your shift.

Exercise outdoors – This will be like killing two birds with one stone; not only are you getting some great exercise, you also benefit from the sunshine, and the positive energy from the outdoor surroundings.

Try relaxing forms of exercise – If you do not like rigorous sports then probably yoga, tai chi, or even just mindful walking might be the right choice for you. Not only will you relieve stress by doing these exercises, these will also teach you to control your impulses and help you to focus much better.

Get Plenty of Sleep Every Day

There is nothing that can worsen the symptoms of adult ADHD more than not getting enough sleep. When you are sleep deprived, your ability to handle stress and focus on tasks will be severely impaired. Thankfully, doing a bit of tweaking to your daytime habits goes a long way towards making sure that you have a good night's sleep.

Here are some of the changes that you need to integrate into your daily habits so you will not have any problem falling asleep at night:

- Do not take any form of caffeine late in the day. Cut yourself off from coffee by 4PM so that your body will have more than enough time to process the caffeine in your system and eliminate it completely by the time you hit the sack.

- Do not exercise an hour before your bedtime. You will be so wired because of the amount of adrenaline coursing through your veins that you will have trouble falling asleep later.

- Form a quiet "bedtime" routine that will help you relax. Choose activities that are quiet and predictable, like taking a hot shower before bed, drinking a warm glass of milk, and maybe reading a couple of pages of your favorite book.

- Stick to a regular sleep-wake schedule. Do not sleep in or stay up late during the weekends or the holidays. Always wake up and go to bed at the same time every day so that your body will get used to the routine.

- Eat healthy. Do not binge eat during dinnertime. You need let your body rest during the night, and this includes your digestive system. Also, try to eat more fruits and vegetables so that you will not experience any vitamin or nutrient deficiencies that could further exacerbate your ADHD.

- If you can, completely eliminate sugar and junk foods from your diet.

Practice Mindfulness

Mindfulness meditation is not just for reducing stress. You can also use it to train yourself to resist distractions, decrease your impulsivity, improve your focus, and to better control your emotions.

Since meditating will require you to sit still for a period of time, having ADHD can make this feel like torture, which is why you need to start slow and work your way up. Meditate for just a short time initially, like say five minutes every day for a week, and then increase the time to ten minutes the next week. The more you become comfortable with the process, the longer you will be able to maintain your focus.

You just then need to draw on what you learned from your mindfulness meditation sessions and apply them into your daily life to keep yourself on track towards a normal, productive life.

You can try meditating on your own, or you can join classes that teach these techniques. Alternatively, you can use free smartphone apps or online videos of guided meditations which makes things a whole lot easier.

Chapter 6 – Understanding Your Loved One's ADHD

Being in a relationship with someone who has ADHD can feel like a constant struggle; a lot of the time you might feel lonely, unappreciated, and maybe even ignored. You may begin to feel tired of being the one who has to take care of everything and grow tired of feeling like the only one who is responsible. You may not feel like you can rely on your partner for anything. It can feel as if your significant other just does not care anymore.

It is plain to see just how both sides of the relationship contribute to its own destruction because one of them has ADHD; the partner without ADHD often complains a lot, nags, and becomes resentful over time, while the one with ADHD feels as if they are constantly being judged, will get defensive, and pull away from the relationship. However, it does not have to be this way, both parties could be happy with the relationship, even with the ADHD. There are many ways that you can face the challenges presented by ADHD, and you will learn how to communicate better, thus becoming more understanding of your partner and more accepting of their condition. It really all begins with understanding how ADHD affects your partner, and the challenges that they face as a result.

What is the role of ADHD in Relationships?

If you want to transform your relationship, you need to start by understanding ADHD's role in it. The moment you learn to identify how ADHD's symptoms are affecting not just your partner, but you as well, you will start to learn better ways to respond. For the partner with ADHD, this means learning to manage your symptoms better, and for the non-ADHD partner, it means learning to react to your frustrations in such a way that it actually encourages your partner to try harder.

Practicing Empathy

The first, and one of the most important steps in improving your relationship is trying to see things through your partner's eyes.

Do not think that just because the two of you have been together for a long time, that you already know where your partner is coming from. You should never underestimate just how easy it is to misinterpret the actions of your partner and their attached intentions. You and your partner are quite different from each other, especially if you are not the one who has ADHD.

The best way to empathize with someone is to just ask and wholeheartedly listen to the answers. Make time to just sit down and talk, preferably when you are not yet upset at your partner. Let your partner tell you just how they feel; do not interject to defend yourself or explain your viewpoint. After your partner has finished talking, repeat the main points that you heard so far, and ask if what you understood about them is right. Writing down the points made by your partner will allow you to reflect on them later.

After your partner has finished airing their grievances, then it is your turn to talk. Ask your partner to do the same for you.

How to Increase the Empathy in Your Relationship?

Study ADHD - It is not enough that your partner alone understands their own condition, you should also study up on ADHD yourself so you will know what you are dealing with. When you learn about how ADHD affects people, you might experience a "Eureka!" moment. Almost all of your relationship issues may suddenly make sense! Once you know that the brain of a person with ADHD is wired differently than that of a normal person, you will start to understand why your partner is acting peculiarly, and you will learn not to take the behavior personally.

Acknowledge how your behavior affects your partner – If you are the one with ADHD, you need to recognize just how your untreated symptoms are affecting your partner. If you are the non-ADHD partner, consider how bad your partner feels when you constantly nag, and your partner cannot do anything about it, because it is just the way the ADHD-affected brain works.

Separate your partner from their symptoms – Rather than labeling your partner as "irresponsible", you need to recognize that being forgetful and not being able to follow through with tasks are symptoms of ADHD, they are not your partner's character traits. This is the same with the non-ADHD partner; the reason your partner constantly nags and complains is because of frustration, and not because your partner is not loving, they just do not know.

How A Person with ADHD Often Feels

Different from others – The brain of a person with ADHD is constantly racing and full of different thoughts. People with ADHD experience the world differently from others.

Under constant stress – Most adults with ADHD would rather not have to deal with their symptoms, mainly because it can be a constant struggle just to get by. Doing mundane tasks takes a lot more mental energy than what normal people use. Finishing simple tasks will require so much concentration that they feel exhausted afterwards.

Subordinate to their spouses – People with ADHD often feel inferior to their spouses, mainly because they are always corrected, reminded, and pushed around. Many men with ADHD report feeling emasculated because they are often scolded.

Ashamed – People with ADHD often hide behind a humorous façade so other people cannot see the huge amount of shame that they are feeling because of their "incompetence".

Unloved and unwanted – The constant reminders they get from their spouses, bosses, and other people that they should "change" and become more responsible only reinforce the idea in their head that they are incompetent and undeserving of love.

Afraid of failing over and over – People with ADHD often sadly set low expectations for themselves because they already anticipate failure. In many ADHD sufferer's minds, they are already a failure before they try.

Longing to be accepted – One of the strongest, if not the strongest emotion that is in people with ADHD is their wanting to be loved and accepted in spite of their flaws. This is the result of years of being talked down to.

How The Non-ADHD Partner Often Feels

Unwanted/unloved – The lack of attention is often misinterpreted as lack of interest, but the truth is that the partner with ADHD is just often distracted.

Angry – Anger and resentment are often included with every interaction with the spouse with ADHD. And because they are sick and tired of angry interactions, the non-ADHD spouse often will keep their feelings bottled up inside of them, which is a very unhealthy practice.

Stressed out of their minds – The spouse without ADHD often carries the bulk of the burden of running the household, so they cannot let their guard down even for a moment. They have to compensate for their ADHD spouse's lack of consistency, or else their entire family will suffer.

Ignored – The non-ADHD spouse can take offense when the ADHD spouse does not act on the example the non-ADHD spouse sets, and doesn't follow the advice the non-ADHD spouse gives, even though it is very "clear" what needs to be done.

Take Responsibility for Your Role

When you can empathize with your spouse, you can then begin to accept responsibility for your role in your relationship. Things will start to get better once you are aware of your own contributions to the ongoing problems that your relationship has, and the same goes for the non-ADHD partner as well.

Even though it is the ADHD partner's symptoms that serve as a trigger for issues, they are not the only ones to blame for the problems. The way that the non-ADHD partner reacts to the symptoms of ADHD can either serve as a doorway for cooperation and compromise, or it could provoke even more conflicts and misunderstandings. If you are the one with ADHD, be mindful of how you react to your partner's reactions; your actions will either validate or disregard the feelings of your spouse, so be careful.

Free Yourselves from the Parent-Child Dynamic

Many couples feel as if they are in an unsatisfying, and sometimes embarrassing, parent-child type of a relationship, with the non-ADHD spouse always taking care of the one with ADHD. This often starts when the spouse with ADHD starts to forget to follow through with daily tasks, like forgetting to pick up the kids after school, or leaving piles of dirty plates in the sink. The non-ADHD partner will start to take on more of the household tasks.

The more lopsided the relationship becomes, the more resentful the non-ADHD spouse feels. Even if the ADHD spouse manages to do something good for a change and actually contributes, the non-ADHD spouse may easily brush them off. Of course, the ADHD spouse will feel this resentment, and will start to feel as if nothing will ever please the non-ADHD spouse. This is an unhealthy dynamic in relationships, and you need to break this before it worsens.

Tips for the non-ADHD spouse/partner

You cannot dictate the actions of your spouse, but you do have control over yours. You should make an effort to stop verbally attacking and nagging your partner as this never produces positive results.

Recognize and congratulate your partner when they make any kind of progress and acknowledge all achievements and efforts.

Whenever possible, focus on your partner's intentions for doing something, not the results that your partner gets. For instance, your partner's mind might start to drift away while you are having a conversation, but that does not mean your partner does not care about what you were trying to say.

Stop trying to become a "parent" to your partner. Not only will doing so demotivate your spouse, doing so can also hurt your relationship.

Tips for the Partner with ADHD

Acknowledge that your ADHD symptoms have put a dent on your relationship. It is not just because your spouse is being unreasonable or not being understanding enough.

Actively look for treatment options. Do not deny that you have ADHD. The sooner that you accept your condition, the sooner you can get treatments to control your symptoms, which will make your and your spouse's life a whole lot easier.

If, during a conversation, you feel as if you are starting to lose control of your emotions, ask for a time out so that you can calm down and refocus. The two of you need to agree to this kind of setup in advance.

Actively find ways to spoil your spouse. If your spouse feels spoiled, even in small peculiar ways, they will feel less like a parent and more like a partner.

Cease Fighting and Commence Communication

As you may already have experienced firsthand, when one spouse has ADHD, effective communication is often very difficult. One partner feels overburdened with responsibilities, while the other feels attacked. So, instead of talking to solve issues, they end up fighting.

One of the best ways to improve communication is to defuse emotional volatility as much as you can. If needed, take a break to cool your heads before you discuss any kind of issue. When you do have a conversation, do your best to listen intently to your partner. You need to ask yourself what the cause of the argument is.

Do not keep your emotions bottled up inside of you. You need to always let your feelings known, regardless of how ugly it might turn things. You need to get your issues out in the open so the two of you can work things through.

You should not make any assumptions about what your spouse is thinking, and most of all, do not doubt your spouse's love for you. If your spouse did something that made you feel upset, address it immediately, and do not let it stew inside of you.

Watch your words and your tone. People who have undiagnosed ADHD know that they have shortcomings, but they often struggle to change on their own, so they are easily triggered when you say something that is critical of their person. Avoid critical statements that will only put your partner on the defensive, like "Why can't you ever do that thing that you always said you would?" or "How many times do I have to repeat myself until you learn?"

Learn to laugh at yourselves. Miscommunications and misunderstandings are inevitable, so why not just find the humor in the situation. Nothing can relieve the tension in the air better than laughter.

How to Improve Your Communication Skills When You Have ADHD?

The symptoms that come with ADHD can also interfere with the way you communicate. The good thing here is that there are some things you can do to improve the way you communicate with your partner and others.

Speak face to face if possible – Spoken words are important in communication, but there are other factors that are at play, like body language, tone of voice, and other gestures that convey important information.

Employ active listening, and do not interrupt – When it is the other person's turn to talk, make a conscious effort to make eye contact and listen to every word. If you catch your mind starting to wander off, mentally repeat the words that you last heard so that you can jog yourself back into listening. Even if you feel a strong urge to interject, do not speak until it is your turn.

Ask questions – Instead of launching into a long rant about the things that have been whirling around your mind or being critical about the things the other person said, just start by asking a question. Not only will you gain more information this way, this will also show the other person that you are actually listening.

Do not be afraid to ask the other person to repeat – When you catch yourself drifting off while you are talking with another person, ask the other person if they could repeat themselves.

Control your emotions – If you are easily triggered when discussing a particular subject, and you let your emotions get the best of you, this can often lead to you saying things that you may regret later. If this happens to you often, then you might want to consider practicing mindfulness meditation. This helps lower your impulsivity, increase focus, and allow you to better control your temper. Being more mindful will help prevent emotional outbursts that can hurt relationships.

Team-up against ADHD – Just because one partner has ADHD, that does not mean that the two of you can't have a fulfilling relationship. You need to work together so that your relationship can work despite of ADHD.

Take a bit of time to identify what each of you are good at, and which tasks pose the biggest challenge. For instance, if your spouse is great at certain tasks that you do not like doing, then perhaps they can take over them instead of you, and vice-versa. You should have equal amounts of tasks so your relationship does not feel lopsided.

Divide your tasks and stick to them – The non-ADHD partner will likely be more suitable for handling the bills and running errands, while the other may be better suited to watching over the kids, and cooking, for example.

Schedule weekly family meetings – You should sit down and discuss the progress that the two of you have made so far, as well as any issues that arose in the relationship during the week.

Delegate, outsource, and automate – The two of you might not be the only ones that have to deal with household tasks. If you have children, put them to work on tasks that they can do. You might also want to hire a nanny to help look after the kids while you work or sign up for a weekly cleaning service. You could also begin using grocery delivery apps so you do not have to leave the house, and automating your bill payments.

Step in to help if necessary – If the partner with ADHD is visibly struggling to finish an assigned task, the non-ADHD partner might need to swoop in to help. You need to take into this into consideration so that resentments can be avoided.

Create a Practical Plan of Action

If you are the one struggling with ADHD, then organizing or setting up systems is probably not your forte. But that does not mean you cannot follow a plan once it is in place; this is where the non-ADHD partner can help. They can assist you in putting in place a system and routine that will help you stay on top of your responsibilities.

Begin by thinking back on the things that you usually fight about, such as unfinished chores, or chronic forgetfulness. Then, think about the practical things that the two of you can do to solve these problems. For instance, for the unfinished chores, you could hang a huge calendar on your wall with checkboxes next to the person's assigned tasks. The calendar will serve as a constant reminder for the ADHD partner to finish their chores.

Helping Your Partner with ADHD

Help your partner develop routines – Having a routine can help people with ADHD because they will benefit from having a bit of structure in their lives. You need to create schedules for the tasks that the both of you have to accomplish, and also factor in time for having meals, exercise, and sleep.

Make use of external reminders – You can use a large dry erase board hung on the wall, sticky notes, or a to-do list written on your phone.

Help to get rid of clutter – People with ADHD have a hard time getting themselves organized, and clutter only makes the problem worse. Keeping your home neat and organized can greatly help to minimize distractions around the house.

Conclusion

Thanks again for taking the time to read this book!

You should now have a good understanding of adult ADHD, and the different treatment options that are available. Remember, this book is not intended to serve as medical advice, but rather, as an informative guide to ADHD. Always consult with a medical professional before creating any treatment plan or taking any medication.

I hope you have found this book to be helpful and would like to wish you the best of luck in managing your ADHD!

If you enjoyed this book, please take the time to leave me a review on Amazon. I appreciate your honest feedback, and it really helps me to continue producing high quality books.